# JOURNEYS
## *in* Postgraduate
## Medical Education

First published 2011
by Third Space Press
7 Bermondsey Street, London SE1 2DD

A CIP catalogue record is available for this book from the British Library

ISBN 978-0-9556014-7-7

Design: Wilson Hui
Cover image: Alex Josephy

Printed in the UK by Webmart UK Ltd.

# JOURNEYS
## *in* Postgraduate
## Medical Education

Editors
Zoë Playdon
Alex Josephy

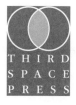

THIRD
SPACE
PRESS

# CONTENTS

# Acknowledgements

As teachers, who should we acknowledge first but our learners, whose desire to learn calls us to teach, and thereby to learn ourselves? So, both learner and teacher create between them a third space, the professional conversation, where we both seek to know more about the values and ideas that we hold in common, the *vertu* that education and medicine both seek to serve. Our especial thanks, then, go to the doctors who have invited us to be guests in their worlds of real-life, problematic, complex clinical practice, and who have accompanied us on our journeys in postgraduate medical education. Similarly, our gratitude is no less to the colleagues who have travelled with us to make this book, both those in KSS Education Department Professional Services, and those involved directly in production. Then, too, we are researchers who, like Renaissance artists, are reliant on our Medici for funding our work, and for being appreciative patrons of our artistry, and so we must register our great appreciation to our CEO, Professor David Black, and to NHS South East Coast, for supporting the educational innovations that we discuss here. Above all, though, we wish to acknowledge the primacy of the patient. We say, good teaching makes best patient care, and it is our absolute purpose, in all our work, that the greatest beneficiary should be the patient population, attended every day by the doctors in KSS.

# Foreword

At a time when postgraduate medical education [PGME] is increasingly under discussion, and subject to change, this book is a unique and timely addition to the developing body of literature on the theory and practice of education, and educational governance, in clinical settings. With its clear explanation of conceptual and educational frameworks, followed by chapters on some of the most exciting developments in the field, drawn from the work of the Kent, Surrey and Sussex Postgraduate Medical Deanery [KSS] in the South East of England, the book provides critical reading, both for those engaged in PGME and, more widely, for students and academics with an interest in contemporary issues in education.

My own journey into PGME has, in some ways, been unusual. I started with a strong interest in management and clinical governance, which led me to think about the different professional roles that make up a NHS hospital consultant's job: teaching, appraisal, management, and so on. Like most clinicians, I learned to teach in an experiential way, and in those days we saw education as 'just part of the job'; there was no talk about the curriculum, or structure, of PGME. Becoming a Medical Director in the 1990s, one of my first priorities was to develop a view of the wider professional needs of the local consultant body, especially those of new consultants, and to put in place a plan to support them. One early decision was that the Trust should require all consultants, including myself, to take the Certificate in Teaching (now QESP Part 1), so that those teaching would have evidence that they could do this to at least a satisfactory standard. This interest still informs my work today as Dean Director at KSS. Chapters 4 to 7 in this book give an account of the course, its unique workplace-based, one-to-one approach, its further development, and the MA programme that has grown out of the department's original work.

I see the innovative work of the KSS Education Department as fulfilling a crucial role in the way in which we ensure high-quality teaching and supervision, and effective implementation of curricula in our region. An intervention of particular note has been the establishment of Local Faculty Groups [LFGs], and a supporting structure to help them to become really useful and effective as the local driver and governance of medical education, as described in Chapter 3.

*Journeys in Postgraduate Medical Education* contains a selection of accounts that takes in topics ranging from educational governance, to a 'community of practice' approach to medical simulation, to the establishment of new approaches to careers guidance. Too often, education is seen as peripheral or, at best, as an entity separate from service, the really important work. My hope for the future is that our work here in KSS will contribute to a shift in PGME, through which all staff and providers will perceive the education of heathcare staff for the future as a core role, intrinsic to high-quality service and high-quality patient care. I recommend this book wholeheartedly to all those interested in education.

David Black
KSS Dean Director
January 2011

# Preface

This book arises from the pioneering work of the Education Department at the Kent, Surrey and Sussex Postgraduate Medical Deanery [KSS] where, for eighteen years, a group of non-clinical academics, whose diverse backgrounds are principally educational, have worked in partnership with medical doctors, in their real-life clinical contexts, to improve education and patient care.

We hope that the chapters that follow might interest other professionals involved in the fast-changing field of medical education, and also those with a wider interest in educational principles and practice, and in understanding the nature of learning and teaching, particularly in the context of adult, work-based learning.

In the first section of our book, we present an account of the current structures, roles, and national initiatives in postgraduate medical education [PGME]. This is followed by an explanation of the Education Department's development, and our underpinning principles, and an account of the process consultancy approach that we adopted to support the local implementation of new, national curriculum frameworks for PGME. In the second section, we focus on a small selection of our activities, presenting some of the ways in which our programmes are organised, linking each of these to specific educational principles, and reflecting from our particular, liminal position on current developments in the field of PGME. The chapters on careers and careers support, on change management, and on working with patients with learning disabilities may also interest readers involved in these areas within other educational contexts. We hope that, in setting down these 'stories that change in the telling', we have conveyed something of the nature and fascination of this work, and its evolving practices.


Alex Josephy
January 2011

# Contributors

### Alex Josephy BA(Hons), PGCE, MA

Alex is an Assistant Dean Education at KSS. As well as having developed the KSS Co-Mentoring programme, and contributing to the development of the Qualified Educational Supervisor Programme, Alex leads on the MA Education in Clinical Settings. A well-published poet as well as an academic, Alex won second prize in the NHS category of the 2010 Hippocrates Awards, for her poem *The Corridor*. Her current interests lie in the use of personal story and organisational narrative as a means of enabling educational change.

### Alison Gisvold PPS, MEd, FRSA, FIfL, MCMI

Alison is an Assistant Dean Education at KSS. She leads on the Supporting Patients with Learning Disabilities and the Co-Mentoring programmes as well as contributing to the Qualified Educational Supervisor Programme and to the School of Leadership. With a former career in the corporate world in the UK and overseas, Alison has lived in Norway for many years, where she published in the area of Entrepreneurship and Language Studies. She is a Fellow of the RSA and the Institute for Learning and a Member of the Chartered Management Institute. Her current interests include researching which leadership styles enable organisations to thrive in periods of economic, social and cultural turbulence; and continuing to promote the rights of individuals with learning disabilities

### Clare Penlington Dip T, BEd, MEd, PhD

Clare is Deputy Head of Academic Programmes and Academic Head of the School of Clinical Leadership at KSS. She has extensive experience in teaching and in educational research. Clare has a particular interest in the role of practitioner research in developing practice, and the way the clinical leadership movement marks a cultural shift in the NHS.

### Joan Reid MBA, FCIPD, M/AGCAS, MAC

Joan is Head of Careers at KSS where she leads the medical careers support team. She is currently completing a Doctorate in Coaching and Mentoring, inquiring into the ways in which coaching supports doctors to make career choices. Joan is joint author, with Caroline Elton, of *ROADS to Success*, a guide to career support for medical students, postgraduate doctors, and their supervisors, which is now in its third edition. Joan and her team also run the NHS medical careers website on behalf of the Department of Health.

## Pam Shaw Dip Ed, MA (Education), EdD, MA (Organisational Consultancy), FHEA

Pam is Deputy Head of Education at KSS. She has a background in teaching in schools and universities and was formerly an external examiner for MA programmes at the University of Manchester and the University of Swansea. Pam holds a doctorate in Education and Master's degrees in Education and in Consulting to Organisations. As well as facilitating the work of KSS Assistant Deans Education, Pam also works part-time as an organisational consultant and executive coach. She is a Fellow of the Higher Education Academy and a member of CARN and OPUS.

## Rachel Robinson Cert Ed, B Phil, MA in Ed (Applied Linguistics), EdD

Rachel is an Assistant Dean Education at KSS. As well as contributing to the MA in Teaching in Clinical Settings, and to the general work of the department, she is the lead for the Qualified Educational Supervisor Programme. Her research interests include the role of spoken language in learning, and the potential for professional conversations to develop and maintain third spaces between participants. Previously, Rachel worked with Primary and Secondary schoolteachers on several National Educational projects, including the National Oracy Project, with its many publications. Her current interests continue to include the relationship between language (particularly talking and listening) and learning.

## Symon Quy BA(Hons), PGCE, MA, MEd, FHEA

Symon is an Assistant Dean Education at KSS. His research interests include educational technologies and using media in teaching and learning. Symon was awarded a National Teaching Fellowship by the Higher Education Academy in 2005 in recognition of his work within Higher Education. Symon is author of *Teaching Short Film* (BFI, 2007) and *Splice Short Film* (Auteur, 2010) and has published widely on media in education. His current interests include supporting Postgraduate Doctor Representatives and empowering Lay Representatives. He leads on Simulation at KSS.

## Zoë Playdon BA(Hons), PGCE, MA, PhD, MEd, DBA, FRSA

Zoë is Professor, Head of Education, and academic lead at KSS. She is particularly interested in the relationship between individual development and organisational change and is the author of books on business planning and on participative management. Formerly Head of Continuing Vocational Education at the University of Warwick, Zoë has senior management experience in compulsory, further and higher education, at local, regional and national levels. Her current research is into integrated medicine and its implications for PGME and patient safety in diverse healthcare communities.

# Part One:

## Principles and Contexts

# National Policy, KSS Strategy and Local Responses

## Postgraduate Doctors

When medical students graduate, they enter postgraduate medical education [PGME] automatically, as an entitlement, for a period of seven to ten years. During their PGME they work and learn in the real-life, everyday setting of clinical care, moving between different hospitals, general practices, and other local education providers [LEPs], including universities.

The first two years of PGME is a Foundation Programme [Foundation]. This is a safe, well-supervised environment, in which these new, postgraduate doctors spend four months in each of six different clinical specialties. Here they learn how to put into practice the principally factual knowledge, or 'propositional knowledge' as it is known, that they gained at medical school. During Foundation, too, they gain a broad understanding of how different specialties interrelate; how primary and secondary care work together; what kinds of careers they might enjoy following; and, crucially, the ethical requirements of good medical practice that must operate in every specialty and in every clinical location. If, at the end of their first year of PGME, they have met the specific requirements laid down by the General Medical Council [GMC], they will be admitted to its Register, and they will now be doctors, very new to the profession, but able independently to manage a patient (GMC 2009).

In the second year of Foundation, postgraduate doctors will be expected to demonstrate increasing sophistication in their clinical skills; in the use of evidence and data; in team-working; and in the reflective insight required to respond well in complex, often highly pressured, high-stakes situations. For the whole of their Foundation, postgraduate doctors maintain a portfolio of achievement to demonstrate their progress in clinical skills and professional development, a practice which they will continue for the rest of their PGME and, indeed, for the whole of their professional careers. Foundation is intended to provide not only a basis for clinical skills and career choice, but also a basis for a set of principles, values, and ethical practices that will provide both a demonstration of, and a touchstone for, their developing understandings as doctors over a lifetime of work.

A period of three to seven years of PGME follows Foundation, leading to a Certificate of Completion of Training [CCT] for General Practice and for hospital medicine respectively. National curriculum frameworks [NCFs] for each specialty are provided by the medical Royal Colleges [Royal Colleges], who also constitute the examinations board for the professional accreditation of PGME. Some specialties operate as 'run-through' programmes, so that following Foundation, entry to the first year is entry to the whole three- or seven-year programme, which concludes with CCT. Other specialties have 'uncoupled' programmes, which provide two or three years of Core Specialty Training [CST], followed by open competition for a further period of Higher Specialty Training [HST], and concluding with CCT. These differing structures illustrate a fundamental principle of PGME: while it is homogenous in its ethical standards, often expressed as its focus on providing best patient care, it is also a massively diverse discipline, covering seventy-four different specialties. The people homogenised in general parlance as 'doctors', like those homogenised as 'academics', are individually representative of a huge range of different knowledge bases, interests, and working circumstances. What is more, doctors, like academics, stand at the intersection of a wide range of social, scientific, legal, and technological change, to which they contribute, and from which they draw.

## The Deanery

This complex system, in which work and learning are inextricably intertwined, is managed regionally by Postgraduate Medical Deaneries [Deaneries]. In some shape or form, Deaneries have been in existence since the inception of the National Health Service [NHS]. In 1944 the Goodenough Report called for 'each university to depute a person to undertake the organisation and general supervision of the postgraduate arrangements' for medical education (Goodenough 1944). In 1968 a Royal Commission, led by Lord Todd, advocated the creation of a national Central Council to exercise strategic oversight, operating through regional committees, with a network of postgraduate medical centres at local level (Todd 1968). The need for robust and effective management of PGME, as part of medicine's professional self-regulation, was highlighted by a Committee of Inquiry in 1975 (Merrison 1975), although by 1988 a King's Fund seminar for postgraduate medical deans, focusing on the need to develop an independent, national authority for PGME, noted that 'the key word was disharmony – between service and educational interests, between medical specialties, between colleges and universities, between regional committees and central bodies – a cacophony of discordant sound' (Parry 1988, 5-6).

Seventeen years later, in 2005, the development of PGME was consolidated by the creation of the Postgraduate Medical Education and Training Board [PMETB], a statutory body, independent of government and nationally responsible for post-registration PGME. In 2009 PMETB amalgamated with the GMC to form a single, overarching body with authority for quality-assuring the whole of PGME. This important step succeeded a period of intense, wide-reaching reforms which had gradually harmonised the 'cacophony'. Following a series of management reforms in the wider NHS, the Calman Report of 1993 introduced planned and structured specialist PGME, managed by Deaneries in collaboration with Royal Colleges. It was decided that the period of time which individuals could spend achieving CCT should be capped rather than unlimited. A new set of NCFs for Foundation and for specialties was developed by Deaneries and Royal Colleges working together with two new national bodies: the United Kingdom Foundation Programme Office [UKFPO] and Modernising Medical Careers [MMC]. Deaneries became responsible for the whole of PGME, for the budgets that fund it, and, under the auspices of the GMC, for quality-managing its provision. In England, quality management for PGME is now carried out by fourteen Deaneries, and in Scotland, Wales and Northern Ireland this service is provided by equivalent bodies, while there is a separate UK Defence Postgraduate Deanery for the armed forces. Most recently, in England, a new body – Medical Education England [MEE] – was created in 2008 as an independent advisory Non-Departmental Public Body [NDPB], to supervise the provision of PGME and to advise Ministers on policy.

Essentially, Deaneries have two main functions: Medical Workforce Management [Medical Workforce] and Education. Medical Workforce combines the function that in mainstream higher education is called 'Admissions' – the processes of selection and recruitment of medical school graduates into PGME – with the management of postgraduate doctors' progression from one LEP to another throughout their education. Unlike in mainstream higher education, however, recruitment to PGME is not only recruitment to education, but also to employment. Half of the doctors in any hospital are postgraduates following their PGME, with the other half – consultants and others in the career grades – providing the faculty that teaches and supervises them in the workplace. Further, postgraduate doctors must move from location to location in order to gain exposure to the range of clinical contexts and cases that are required by their curricula. It is a complex series of rotations between different hospitals, general practices, medical schools, Primary Care Trusts [PCTs], and other LEPs. At the same time, clinical services have to be maintained twenty-four hours a day, seven days a week, all year round, so it must always be the case that enough doctors of the right grade and specialty are present in every clinical setting throughout the region. As an added complication, work and recruitment patterns are subject to changes arising from new legislation, such as the European Working Time Regulations [EWTR]; to changes in demography, so that, for example, Britain's ageing population will eventually require more doctors with expertise in elderly medicine; and to changes in government policy, so that, for instance, a greater emphasis on primary care means an increased need for general practitioners [GPs]. Finally, postgraduate doctors themselves may prefer one career path to another, or may change direction, or move to a different part of the profession, thus creating patterns of supply and demand that have to be managed as part of the Deanery's Medical Workforce role.

Education is the other function of Deaneries, and it is no less complex or less specialist a role than that of Medical Workforce. Automatically, every consultant in every hospital has a teaching role as an intrinsic part of their appointment. This is in contrast to General Practice, in which GPs must choose to apply to become GP Educators. For example, in Kent, Surrey and Sussex Postgraduate Medical Deanery [KSS], this means there are approximately 2,500 consultant educators, in twelve acute and three psychiatric NHS Trusts, spread across the region's healthcare economies. Traditionally, these consultant educators were not required to receive training to become teachers or Educational Supervisors, yet they always carried out this role. They were teaching not just in formal lectures or workshops, but in real-life clinical settings, on ward-rounds, in theatres, and in clinics, whether modelling good practice by their own example, or discussing clinical cases and their treatment with postgraduate doctors. In 2007, however, PMETB (now the GMC) set out a new agenda for every consultant to be educated and accredited as a teacher and as an Educational Supervisor, to standards published in July 2008, with a deadline of January 2010 for completion of the initiative. The GMC's very reasonable requirement is that postgraduate doctors should receive a level of teaching and educational supervision appropriate to their grade, specialty, and the patients they treat. For many Deaneries, however, the rapid timescale provided a logistical problem, as there are no 'out of term' times that might be utilised for teacher education, and the removal of consultants from the workplace has an immediate knock-on effect on their NHS Trust's clinical targets. In KSS our response was to create the work-based Qualified Educational Supervisor Programme [QESP], in which senior educational experts work on a one-to-one basis with clinicians in their real-life clinical setting to develop their teaching while providing as little disruption as possible to the usual provision of patient care.

Educational quality management provides a similar complexity. Traditionally, doctors have learned by a process usually referred to as 'apprenticeship'. In 1993, there was no top limit to the duration of PGME, and individuals spent time moving between different specialties, typically taking PGME-associated jobs at Senior House Officer [SHO] level, until they found the specialty they preferred. They would then look for posts at higher levels, taking examinations as they went, until they were eligible to apply for a consultant post. For many specialties, the NCF was inferred from practice and did not exist as an explicit statement of expectations and boundaries. It could easily take twelve to fourteen years or more before individuals were considered suitable for a consultant post. Further, there was no practical limitation on the number of hours that could be worked, providing access to huge opportunities for experience on the one hand, but opportunities for ruthless exploitation on the other. Progression was a matter of being signed-off at the end of the job, which meant achieving a standard of work that was not explicitly stated or nationally agreed. Because there were no formal standards, being signed-off meant, at worst, complying with the unreasonable whims and demands of the supervising consultant. There was no explicit standard for comparability between individuals or posts, making recruitment from one level of PGME to another an onerous and uncertain process. Interestingly, at the time of writing a similarly traditional situation still exists in undergraduate medicine: unlike other academic disciplines, UK medical schools do not use a uniform process of grading medical degrees.

From 1993 onwards, the series of reforms and innovations initiated by the Calman Report in effect established Deaneries as regional postgraduate academic structures. Deaneries were charged with managing and leading the implementation of new curricula for postgraduate doctors; setting new standards for teacher education for consultants; implementing new processes for ensuring the existence of a sufficient educational infrastructure at LEPs; and establishing new systems for evaluating, controlling and quality-managing the education and assessment of every postgraduate doctor in their region. This meant that KSS, as a medium- to large-sized Deanery, became responsible for managing the learning of approximately 2,500 postgraduate doctors; the teacher education of an equivalent number of teachers and Educational Supervisors; the development of infrastructure in its LEPs; the implementation of new Regional Schools to take forward the new NCFs for each clinical specialty; and the direct development and implementation of new curriculum initiatives in Medical Careers, in Clinical Leadership, and in Simulation. These were not entirely new requirements of course, and all Deaneries had a basis in most of these areas, on which they could build. But the scale of change in its range, depth, and speed, had a character more of revolution than evolution, and of re-engineering rather than progressive development. And of course, there was a strong and immediate knock-on effect for LEPs, especially NHS Trusts.

## LEPs and Local Faculty

Unlike in mainstream higher education, where universities employ the academic staff who teach and research on their behalf, the consultants who teach PGME are not employed by the Deanery, even though the Deanery quality-manages their programmes, their learners, their infrastructure, and their teacher education. Consultants are employed by their NHS Trust, which chooses to accept a contract from the Deanery to provide PGME of a specified standard in return for funding for 50% of the basic salary of the postgraduate doctors who form half of their medical workforce. However, the two key people who head up the local provision of PGME in NHS Trusts, the Director of Medical Education [DME] and the Medical Education Manager [MEM] are jointly appointed by the NHS Trust and the Deanery and as such, they and their teams are local representatives of the Deanery.

DMEs are uniformly senior clinicians, working as part of a clinical team for one part of the week and carrying out their educational leadership role for the other part of the week. MEMs are uniformly non-clinicians, working full-time as specialist senior managers of a crucially important element of the NHS Trust's infrastructure. In the end, the business of an NHS Trust hangs off its doctors, and as half of them are postgraduates, the quality and management of their PGME can have a significant effect on the quality of patient care and on quantitative patient targets for throughput, and for clinical governance. The DME role is to provide leadership and accountability for PGME locally, a role that is usually combined with local responsibility for consultant Continuous Professional Development [CPD], undergraduate medical education, and non-consultant career-grade CPD. Essentially, the DME leads the local faculty; provides accountability for the quality of PGME locally to both the Deanery and the NHS Trust Chief Executive; and co-ordinates the implementation of new educational initiatives across the NHS Trust and across the general practices which provide important curriculum elements to the programmes of all KSS postgraduate doctors.

DMEs are supported by the MEM, whose team typically combines the functions of business management of the local Education Centre, Academic Registrar for PGME locally, and local co-ordination of Medical Workforce. Each NHS Trust contains an Education Centre: many of these were built originally by subscription from the hospital's consultants, but in KSS they are now uniformly multi-professional Education Centres, used by staff from across the whole NHS Trust. Almost all Education Centres include a lecture theatre, seminar rooms, administrative offices, a café facility, and the NHS Trust Library and Knowledge Services [LKS]. Staffed by specialist, professional Library Service Managers [LSMs], the LKS provide the whole of the NHS Trust's clinical and educational library and knowledge services. LSMs are wholly appointed and work entirely for their NHS Trust. However, the regional LKS team, which forms part of the Education Department at KSS, assists the NHS Trust in appointing the LSMs, involves LSMs in cross-regional and national initiatives, and manages the implementation of region-wide library and knowledge service initiatives.

It is usual for LSMs and MEMs to be line-managed by the DME, since it is their effective joint working that makes or breaks PGME locally, and thereby improves or disadvantages clinical services. All three of these roles have changed and developed as new responsibilities, curricula, standards, and systems have been introduced nationally. In KSS, we have sought to work collaboratively with DMEs, MEMs, and LSMs to create new systems to support local implementation of new developments. In particular, both KSS and its NHS Trusts have worked hard to ensure that the local educational infrastructure is as good as it can be, through the annual process of quality manual verification, education strategic planning, and agreement of targets which we call 'Contract Review'. More recently, with the introduction of new NCFs and the national educational standards and aspirations for PGME that they embody, we have worked jointly to create a system of Local Faculty Groups [LFGs]. Where an individual Royal College is responsible for producing the NCF for its specialty – Anaesthetics, for instance – the LFG is responsible for creating a Local Curriculum in Practice [LCP] that reflects the learning opportunities available within the LEP. So, an individual LEP will bring together everyone involved in teaching, assessing, and managing Anaesthetics to work as a group to write their LCP for Anaesthetics, which will translate the aspirations and targets of the NCF for Anaesthetics into real-life practice. In KSS, the process for doing this requires each LFG to produce a Student Handbook, describing their LCP, setting out the learners' entitlements and responsibilities, and describing the learning resources available locally. Each LFG meets three times a year to discuss the progress of every learner. Running in parallel with the LFG, postgraduate doctors in each local faculty also meet three times a year to discuss the progress of the teaching they receive, to report on it to the LFG, and to raise queries and suggestions about their local curriculum.

KSS originally created and implemented LFGs in all of its LEPs in 2005, as a means of managing Foundation and initially LFGs reported directly to the Foundation School. As the MMC agenda was implemented successively, and all Royal Colleges began producing NCFs for local implementation, KSS required LEPs to set up LFGs for each specialty. It was evident that each LEP would require a local co-ordination mechanism for its LFGs, all of which were using the same LEP infrastructure for education, for recruitment, for recording learners' progression, for developing learning resources, and for managing funding. Accordingly, in 2008 KSS created and implemented a Local Academic Board [LAB] in each NHS Trust, chaired by the DME, managed by an Academic Registrar, and governed by KSS *Graduate Education and Assessment Regulations* [GEAR]. Because PGME is clinically and financially critical for the business of LEPs, and to ensure swift decision making and strong management engagement, there are key members of the LEP's Senior Management Team [SMT] who are part of the LAB: the Medical Director, the Finance Director, the Director of Human Resources, and the IT Director. The LAB meets three times a year, takes reports from each LFG, problem-solves locally and if necessary refers intractable challenges to the appropriate KSS School for resolution. From the point of view of KSS Heads of School [HoS], this means that both the LFG as a faculty, and the LEP as an organisation, have already resolved challenges, insofar as they can, before they arrive at School level. From the LEP point of view, the system means that they have a high degree of local authority and autonomy, and are thus well placed to develop local flexibility and creativity within the appropriate regional and national guidelines. The participatory process through which LFGs and LABs were devised and put in place throughout KSS is described by Pam Shaw in Chapter 3.

# The Learner

At the heart of this complexity lie the individual postgraduate doctors and their learning. Theirs is predominantly a work-based learning experience, in which they develop their skills, knowledge, and experience through working under the supervision of more senior colleagues. As a group, they represent a new idea of PGME: doctors are taught an explicit, time-based curriculum with regular assessment, they are required to maintain an educational portfolio, and they work to limited hours. This is a radical departure for medicine and there is considerable concern about the kinds of consultants that this new approach will produce in the future. Certainly, common sense alone suggests that they will have had considerably less exposure to clinical contexts and patient care, and fewer opportunities to experience complex and critical case care, than their forerunners. Consultants of the future will have had less time to decide on their choice of career within medicine. Furthermore, they will have faced greater demands to act as educators and managers while carrying out their clinical roles. In KSS we had provided a level of specialist Careers Support, as a matter of good practice, for seven years before it was introduced officially into the PGME curricula. Consequently we were able to innovate rapidly and to take on a national role in that area, an experience that Joan Reid discusses in Chapter 10.

Other recent, significant developments in the curriculum of postgraduate doctors include Simulation, Clinical Leadership, and Medical Humanities. Simulation offers opportunities to explore clinical circumstances and to develop new skills in a safe environment. It is particularly helpful, for example, for Foundation Year One [F1] postgraduate doctors to be able to simulate stabilising the condition of a very sick patient, and to simulate assisting in diagnosis. These are duties that they are not legally able to carry out in a real clinical situation until they have been admitted to GMC registration. This kind of learning experience, its integration with the curriculum, and the potential for developing dramatic, enacted, 'as if' scenarios, is important in a range of ways. The KSS approach, which we term 'Curriculum-Led Simulation' [CLS], enables postgraduate doctors to develop clinical skills before practising them on patients; provides a means of exploring interactions in clinical teams and with patients, their families, and their carers; and extends teaching into curricular areas that are problematic to learn solely from real-life clinical practice. Symon Quy in Chapter 8 explores the process of developing and implementing CLS in KSS.

Establishing a regional School of Clinical Leadership in 2009 was a new initiative for KSS, but one that chimed well with its educational principles and expertise. In particular, it offers opportunities to problematise the relationship between the ethically charged environments of medicine and education, and the 'bottom-line' business management imperatives of budget-limited clinical organisations. We have also taken the opportunity to explore the integration of the work-based learning [WBL] setting with the higher education institution [HEI] setting, by creating shared curricula and course teams for our new work-based Master's degree in Clinical Leadership. Each KSS LEP that has a postgraduate doctor following the Master's programme has nominated a Leadership Facilitator, whose role is to ensure that the postgraduate doctor gains access to appropriate forums and expertise in the LEP. Leadership Facilitators, who include Chief Executives and Medical Directors, meet regularly as a group to discuss their work and develop their expertise, so that the initiative has the character of Collaborative Action Research. As well, all KSS LEPs have identified Leadership Champions, whose role is to work with their LAB and LFGs to introduce Leadership as a cross-curriculum initiative supported by the KSS work-based Leadership Education Accreditation Programme [LEAP]. To synthesise senior academic expertise with senior clinical experience, in this new curriculum development, the KSS School is jointly led by a Clinical Head and an Academic Head.

Medical Humanities is the newest area of development in PGME, embracing a wide spectrum of approaches to the arts, humanities, and social sciences, as evidenced by the annual conferences provided by the Association for Medical Humanities [AMH]. It is part of the 'KSS tradition' to recognise that medicine is both an art and a science, and this is a major part of KSS's rationale for maintaining a specialist Education Department, staffed by non-clinical senior academics. Their backgrounds in the arts and social sciences strongly support the Department's involvement in Medical Humanities. This involvement was given focus by the most recent edition of *The Gold Guide* (MMC 2010, 110), which requires that, under the heading of Professionalism, 'In addition to medical knowledge and skills, medical professionals should present psychosocial and humanistic qualities such as caring, empathy, humility and compassion, social responsibility and sensitivity to people's culture and beliefs'. Interest in this new discipline is strongly interdisciplinary, and is well represented in both undergraduate and postgraduate medical education, where it occupies a spectrum from 'art for art's sake' to the clear utilitarianism of 'how the humanities can improve your clinical practice'. Our MA Medical Humanities reflects KSS's broad approach: we teach professionalism through humanistic inquiry, and thereby resist the potential binarisation of Medical Humanities into either a *fin de siècle* aestheticism or a reductionist utilitarianism. This approach is discussed by Zoë Playdon in Chapter 11.

Part of the 'new wave' of PGME is an increased focus on the learner's 'voice'. Formerly it was usual for postgraduate doctors to have an end-of-year meeting, when they gave informal feedback on their experience of their local employment and education. Within the formal management of PGME the learners tended to be tokenised or, at worst, to be abjected, that is, to be made voiceless. When they were invited to PGME meetings as a 'representative', the absence of any induction to that role, or formal definition of it, meant that implicitly, they were expected to speak only when formally invited to do so, unlike the rest of the members attending the meeting. If postgraduate doctors had problems with their learning or with their clinical duties then, in the poorest circumstances, they had no formal process for gaining support, no structured, regular, professional conversations about their progress or their needs, and no forum for bringing about change as a group. In the very worst circumstances, their Educational Supervisor might never meet them or, conversely, might be mercilessly bullying and overbearing. Now, however, the GMC has formalised and made national an annual survey of postgraduate doctors' satisfaction with their education, which was developed initially by London Deanery and carried out in both KSS and London Deaneries for some years before it became a national requirement. This is a route towards allowing the collective voice of learners to be heard. At a more local level KSS has implemented workshops for postgraduate doctors who are representatives on LABs, LFGs, and other Deanery forums and committees, as a means of inducting them to new processes, establishing their right to speak, and valorising their voice.

KSS's focus on the learner's voice is matched by a focus on the patient's voice. In Chapter 9 Alison Gisvold discusses some of the problematics facing Patients with Learning Disabilities [PLDs] in their co-construction of a meaningful discourse with their clinicians. Researching, developing and implementing new approaches in this area of work represents a new challenge to KSS, and yet at the same time it is paradigmatic of every clinical encounter, with its abiding questions of access, autonomy, and authenticity.

We regard voice at the individual level, then, to be of particular importance, and especially voice in dialogue, which we term 'the professional conversation', the ongoing discussion of patients, processes, and principles, through which postgraduate doctors learn in real-life clinical settings. We do not conceive of this as a debate – though it is certainly very urgent at times – since one side is not trying to defeat the opinion of the other. Rather, we view it as a joint exploration, in which all parties have a shared, ethical responsibility to explore every option that might contribute to best patient care. The expectation is that, as in an orchestra, each person will play their own part to mutual benefit, without one part of the orchestra seeking to drown out another. However, in the real-life clinical setting a more accurate metaphor for the professional conversation might be an improvised jazz session, in which each player listens to, supports, develops, and responds to each other player. PGME comprises both scheduled formal teaching in lectures and seminars, and opportunistic learning arising from real-life patient care. So, it combines both an ordered, orchestrated approach to formal education with the spontaneity of professional conversations, occurring anywhere – in corridors, in lifts or in clinical areas. The conductor of this orchestra and the jazz singer leading the improvised sessions is a consultant educator, one of the 2,500 senior doctors who provide the faculty for secondary care in KSS.

## The Teacher

General Practice organised its teachers, nationally and regionally, at a much earlier date than was the case in secondary care. Well before the Calman Report, general practices had to go through a rigorous process of approval, and GPs themselves had to undertake structured programmes of teacher education before being allowed to teach postgraduate doctors. By contrast, in 1993 a small group of Accident and Emergency consultants approached KSS's new Head of Education to say that they had been teaching for years, that they had no idea whether they were doing so well or badly, and that they wanted advice. The KSS Certificate in Teaching [CiT] was developed from work with this first group of consultant educators. Over time the CiT developed into QESP, which is discussed by Rachel Robinson and Alex Josephy in Chapters 4, 5 and 6.

In both primary and secondary care, teaching takes place predominantly in the real-life clinical setting through the process of providing medical care. Although there is an important component of lectures, seminars and tutorials, it is the opportunistic teaching that arises from particular patients and their needs, which is foregrounded in real-life practice. Identifying and using these affordances for teaching – the few moments available on a ward-round, perhaps when moving between wards, the preparation time before a procedure is carried out in theatre, or the tiny interval between patient appointments in clinics – to their best effect, is a particularly important aspect of the teacher's role, therefore. KSS teacher education follows this clinical lead, by operating in the real-time clinical settings of theatres, ward-rounds, and clinics, to provide practice-based accreditation of teaching and educational supervision. Taking this to the next level, our MA Education in Clinical Settings focuses on practitioner inquiry into teaching, curriculum, and leading educational change in participants' real-life clinical settings.

With the introduction of new curricula and MMC, KSS teachers have organised themselves into LFGs to co-ordinate their teaching, formalise their assessment processes, manage the progression of their learners, and consider their own development needs as educators. All of them have the opportunity to follow QESP and to develop their capacity for using the professional conversation in teaching in clinical settings, and in their interactions as a LFG. Effectively, they are forming themselves into communities of practice to develop shared boundaries and expectations, and a shared language in which to discuss education. In Chapter 3 Pam Shaw discusses aspects of this 'holding' process for the learner and the LCP.

## The Medical Royal Colleges

In existence many years before the formation of the NHS (the Royal College of Physicians was established in 1518), Royal Colleges are independent bodies that combine the functions of membership organisations and examinations boards. Effectively, they set the standards for the professional accreditation of doctors in each of the seventy-four specialties in the

UK. Deaneries work in close partnership with Royal Colleges, most recently by establishing regional Specialty Schools. These are led by HoS who work for the Deanery, but are appointed jointly with the appropriate Royal College and may also have College duties or appointments. It is the Royal Colleges that create the NCFs for PGME and while it is not technically necessary to pass College examinations in order to achieve CCT, it would be very unusual for postgraduate doctors not to do so.

As well as providing the curriculum standards for postgraduate doctors, Royal Colleges also set the standards for professional revalidation of career-grade doctors, and they support this by providing appropriate CPD opportunities. They have an important independent advisory role – to individual NHS Trusts, to Deaneries, to statutory bodies such as the GMC, and to government. As senior bodies for the professional accreditation of PGME, Royal Colleges are active collaborators with Deaneries and with higher education.

## The Universities

Where the Deaneries and Royal Colleges jointly provide professional accreditation for medicine, the universities provide academic qualification. Central to this, of course, are the medical schools, providing undergraduate and postgraduate qualifications in medical specialties, but, increasingly, their wider university frameworks are being brought into play. The new emphasis on education in medicine has been supported, in many cases, by expertise from university Education Departments, and the new initiative on Clinical Leadership finds natural support in university Business Schools. As well, the small but vigorous and growing interest in Medical Humanities necessarily draws from the arts, humanities, and social science divisions of higher education for its content, rationale, and critique. Finally, universities have long-term experience of collaboration with industry, especially through departments of Continuing Education, technology transfer offices, and consultancy arrangements, and this experience may be helpful to new initiatives in PGME.

In particular, of course, universities are the UK's central locations for research, both pure and applied, in the wide range of subject areas, in the sciences, technologies, social sciences, and humanities that come into play in providing best patient care in the NHS. This is typified by the special relationship that exists between medical schools and the hospitals attached to them, which provide a tertiary level of specialist care, based on the medical school's specialist expertise. In practice, medical schools and the NHS Trusts which are located therein are almost indistinguishable from each other, with clinical academic staff usually jointly appointed, and consultants and academics both working in each other's locations. Inevitably, too, the same staff find themselves providing their specialist expertise to support the work of Royal Colleges, creating yet another organisational cross-over, and ensuring the tight weaving of the clinical fabric of PGME.

## The KSS Education Department

KSS Education Department has worked with the contexts, organisations, and approaches described above since its inception in 1993, on the initiative of one of its Deans, Mr Peter Savage, a consultant surgeon at Queen Mary's Hospital, Sidcup. From the start, the concept was to introduce senior, specialist academic expertise from mainstream education into PGME, to provide a cross-fertilisation of ideas, and thus to develop innovative practice. At the time of writing, nine academic staff are employed in this way, with the Head of Education appointed at the professorial grade. The work of the Department operates to a coherent set of principles and processes called 'a principled approach to practice', which is the subject of the next chapter.

The Department's academic staff members, the 'Assistant Deans Education' [ADEs], are drawn from backgrounds in teacher education and continuing education. Their role is to research, develop, implement, and evaluate innovative solutions to meet the rapidly changing needs of PGME, regionally, locally, and nationally. Part of the task, then, is similar to that of academic staff in mainstream higher education, in that ADEs must be active researchers, in touch with the latest developments in mainstream and in medical education. However, the result of their research is less likely to be publication of academic writing (though that is an important element) and much more the practical development and implementation of innovation. In that sense, therefore, the ADE role is strongly concerned with process management and consultation with organisations and teams. At the same time, ADEs have an important teaching role, providing programmes both for professional accreditation (such as QESP), and for academic qualification up to Master's and Doctoral levels. Further, the Department is responsible for academic quality management for PGME in KSS, leading on quality management of the secondary care LEP educational infrastructure for the Deanery, including producing the Education Contract signed between the Chief Executive Officer [CEO] of NHS Trusts and the Deanery.

During 2008, the Education Department piloted the UK's first academic qualification in Managing Medical Careers (now an MA programme) in collaboration with Brighton and Sussex Medical School [BSMS]. This provides opportunities for LEPs, Deaneries, and Royal Colleges to build specialist Careers teams, combining academic excellence with professionally accredited Careers Advisers. The Education Department was also responsible for brokering the introduction of the UK's Medical Careers Website, in collaboration with the Academy of American Medical Colleges [AAMC], NHS Employers, and MMC, and it now hosts the website on behalf of the Department of Health [DH].

Most recently, the regional LKS team has joined the Education Department. They co-ordinate and develop all of library and knowledge services, for clinical and educational purposes, for the whole of the NHS workforce in KSS, and thus their remit goes far wider than PGME. However, as a research culture grows within LEPs, as closer relationships are formed between local healthcare economies and their universities, and as educational understandings become increasingly sophisticated, development of the capacity of LKS to support these initiatives will be crucial.

At the time of writing, therefore, the Education Department comprises three interrelated functions: Education, LKS and Careers, and it is supported by a professional services team. Internally to the Deanery, it works collaboratively with the Medical Workforce function and especially with the new HoS; externally, it works collaboratively with all of the agencies described above at regional, local, and national levels. In particular, collaborative working at national level is facilitated by the National Education Advisers' Forum [NEAF], a regular forum where UK Deanery Education Advisers meet to exchange and develop their practice. Whether they are working internally or externally, the role of academic staff is the same: to critique, problematise, and analyse the needs of PGME in KSS; to establish a coherent educational philosophy that will underpin new developments to meet those needs; and, drawing on the full range of educational disciplines – history, philosophy, sociology, psychology, leadership, arts and sciences – to create and implement new systems and processes. The nature of our educational philosophy is the subject of the next chapter, while discussion of some of its outcomes forms the remainder of this book.

# References

Committee of Inquiry into the Regulation of the Medical Profession. 1975. *Report*. [Merrison Committee]. Command 6018. London: HMSO.

General Medical Council. 2009. *The New Doctor*. London: GMC.

KSS Education Department. 2010. *GEAR: Graduate Education and Assessment Regulations*. 3rd edition. London: KSS.

Ministry of Health and Department of Health for Scotland. 1944. *Report of an Inter-Departmental Committee on Medical Schools*. [Goodenough Committee]. London: HMSO.

Modernising Medical Careers (MMC). 2010. *A Reference Guide for Postgraduate Specialty Training in the UK: The Gold Guide*. 4th edition. London: NHS.

Parry, K., ed. 1988. *Improving Postgraduate and Continuing Education*. London: King Edward's Hospital Fund for London for the United Kingdom Conference of Postgraduate Deans.

Royal Commission on Medical Education. 1968. *Report* 1965-68. [Todd Committee]. Command 3569. London: HMSO.

# A Principled Approach to Practice: a Practised Approach to Principles

## Meeting-points

Postgraduate medical education [PGME] stands at the confluence of powerful currents in policy, polity, and philosophy. In policy terms, PGME provides a meeting-point for two major areas of government debate and development: Health and Education. Organisationally, the management and governance of PGME is shared by Postgraduate Medical Deaneries [Deaneries], which are public-sector bodies accountable to the NHS, and by medical Royal Colleges [Royal Colleges], which are private-sector bodies long established by Royal Charter. Philosophically, it is axiomatic that medicine is both an art and a science, in which patient interactions bring together evidence-based sciences and empirical observations to inform clinical judgements.

For the practitioner teaching postgraduate doctors in surgeries and theatres, on ward-rounds and domestic visits, in clinics, and outpatients, the most interesting of these three powerful currents perhaps, is the philosophy that underpins their teaching. It is certainly the one that has the most immediate impact on the well-being of their learners and their patients, and one that they have most control over, in that they can inquire into it every day as part of their usual working life. What is more, if a practitioner decides to engage with the politics or the management of PGME, then it is their educational philosophy, anchored in their real-life clinical practice, which will provide keel and compass for navigating these often turbulent environments.

PGME's philosophical inheritance is broad, drawing equally on the great humanistic consciousness rooted in European antiquity and flowering in the Renaissance, and on the complex development of the sciences and social sciences that was fuelled by the Enlightenment. These are living traditions for medicine, so that its contemporary letters and articles in the *British Medical Journal* [BMJ] are as likely to reach backwards to Asklepios and Greek mythology as a touchstone for humanism, as they are to reach forwards to nuclear physics and complexity theory as illumination of new sciences. All of this knowledge is required by PGME, since it teaches professional practice *in practice*, that is by working with patients in the real-life clinical setting.

There, the new empiricism of evidence-based medicine is harnessed to an older empirical tradition of observed cause and effect over time, with both contributing to the patient's and doctor's shared narrative about what is happening, and what should happen next. Fundamentally, the scientific ideal of a single, absolute truth becomes, in practice, a complex drawing together of a series of different truths, to identify a range of options and inform selection from them. Somewhat paradoxically, therefore, scientific data from randomised controlled trials and observational methods are mediated through a humanistic tradition of narrative-based evidence. It is these humanistic and scientific narratives, woven together, which make sense of the information arising from the various sciences and technologies, thereby enabling practitioners to teach their practice, to discuss options with patients, colleagues, and learners, and thus to ensure informed patient consent.

PGME, therefore, is the recipient of wide and varied intellectual traditions, with an inheritance that stretches backwards to earliest times, and a talent for the rapid colonisation and deployment of contemporary scientific and technological discoveries. At the same time, it is highly vulnerable to the winds of political change and competing political agendas, and the checks and balances contributing to its management and provision are many and complex. However, within these complexities, and illuminating a route through them, lies a philosophy – a set of principles and values – that medicine holds as inviolable, and which forms an inalienable patient entitlement. In clinical contexts, these values are expressed as the ethical principles of biomedicine, listed briefly as autonomy, justice, beneficence, and non-maleficence. As it happens, these are the same principles that inform the ethics of education. Teachers, like doctors, work with people who are vulnerable, to whom they have the capacity to do lasting harm, and who, therefore, trust them to be skilful, compassionate helpers. This is true of learners of all ages, as it is of patients of all ages. Thus, teaching, like medicine, is a morally charged activity, and it is through this shared concern with moral lawfulness that Assistant Deans Education [ADEs] enter the world of PGME at Kent, Surrey and Sussex Postgraduate Medical Deanery [KSS].

## KSS Education Department

KSS Education Department was set up in 1993 specifically to bring ideas from mainstream higher education into PGME, with a view to enabling its change and development at local, regional, and national levels. Explicitly, therefore, ADEs stand at an intersection between PGME and university departments of education, actively engaged in creative dialogue with both about practice, principles and processes in education. Fortunately, although there are distinct differences in roles, responsibilities, and regulatory arrangements between the two locations, they are linked by common professional principles and practices. Both PGME and university education operate in real-life settings to support professionals in developing their practice. Both are strongly process-based and focus on working with people to improve their well-being. Fundamental to both is the process of discussion, of sharing ideas and possibilities, in order to find new ways ahead. Crucially, though, both offer processes which can bring about great change to the people with whom they work, either for good or for harm, and thus both PGME and university education foreground a shared set of ethical values. Succinctly, both of them have an explicit rationale that governs their practice, informs their professional debates, and provides the basis for their professional judgements.

It is that rationale, expressed as a set of ethical principles, that KSS ADEs take directly into the real-life, complex, problematic world of PGME, teaching hospital consultants how to teach, in their everyday clinical settings of theatres, wards, and clinics. At the same time, it is the experience of working with consultant educators, in their complicated relationships with patients, learners and colleagues, that shapes and informs those ethical principles, by locating them in specific contexts, as lived experience. Principles and practice are inextricably intertwined, with the one illuminating the other; the intention is that the work of ADEs should be at once a principled approach to practice and a practised approach to principles, with both approaches held in what we term 'the professional conversation'. Aspects of this are explored throughout this book. Crucial to this work, and to our rationale for it – that is, crucial to the KSS philosophy of education – is the relationship between different kinds of knowledge, understood most immediately as the relationship between education and training.

## Education and Training

As the philosopher R. S. Peters (1967, 15, 19) famously points out, the presence or absence of a rationale makes the distinction between education and training:

> The concept of 'training' has application when (i) there is some specifiable type of performance that has to be mastered, (ii) practice is required for the mastery of it, (iii) little emphasis is placed on the underlying rationale.

> The typical term for the educational process by means of which people are brought to understand principles is 'teaching'; for 'teach' unlike 'train' or 'instruct', suggests that a *rationale* is to be grasped behind the skill or body of knowledge.

This distinction is echoed constantly in the literature of education and is a fundamental part of the KSS approach to PGME, where the purpose of making a distinction between education and training is to enable a better understanding of their relationship in practice:

> Where training takes responsibility for the workplace only, education recognises that it must deal with the whole person, that personal and professional life are intertwined. So, instead of requiring people to follow

only instructions, the philosophy of education is to empower learners to take control of and responsibility for their own learning and at the same time to be personally accountable. In real terms this distinction manifests itself in the statement that education contains training but that training cannot contain education (Playdon and Goodsman 1997, 983).

Or, as Barrow and Woods (1988, 18) put it:

The direct implication is that education is really about people developing in certain preferred ways, living lives involving much more than the assimilation of knowledge for the sake of knowledge.

This view of education is echoed by that of Stone (1992, 3) in his work *Quality Teaching*:

Few, surely, would disagree that teachers should have a good grasp of subject knowledge and should be familiar with schools and classrooms. However, the 'delivery' view of teaching grossly oversimplifies its true nature, and the prescriptions intended to improve it are doomed to fail because of the lack of understanding of its complexities.

Stone is reflecting a coherent theme in contemporary educational thinking, inherent in distinctions such as those made between 'knowing how' and 'knowing that' (Ryle 1949, 25-61), or 'technical knowledge' and 'practical knowledge' (Oakeshott 1962, 7-8), or 'practical knowledge' and 'propositional knowledge' (Eraut 1994, 15). A recent, vigorous and well-referenced exposition of these principles as they operate in surgical education is provided by de Cossart and Fish (2005, 39-48).

## Practical Wisdom

It would be easy to see education and training as falling into two opposite camps, defined by their opposition to each other, but to do so would be wrong. In philosophy, as in science, the purpose of making distinctions is to understand the right ordering of relationships, not to create false contraries. No-one supposes that the skeletal and the nervous systems of the body are either the same thing or at odds with each other. Rather, the relationship between education and training is like the relationship between the white and the yolk of an egg, that is, a larger term containing a smaller, distinct term.

So, training, as the yolk of the egg, is typified by a set of instructions that must be adhered to at all times and in all circumstances, for actions that must be performed uniformly, as part of a process that is highly routinised, and as the means to an end which is completely predictable. The need for personal discretion or professional judgement on the part of the individuals, ideally, is reduced to zero: people are trained to act only as operatives in a system that admits no flexibility, no alternative responses, and no creativity. If a learner's question can be answered with the phrase 'Always and only...', then the learner is in a training environment, with its immensely effective, extremely valuable, uniform, fixed systems. Training, therefore, is used in production-line settings, to establish uniform responses and processes across complex systems and environments. It is, so to speak, the bread and butter of professional practice, which ensures that patient information is well handled, clinical equipment works, supplies are ordered, tests are carried out and reported on, and wards are cleaned.

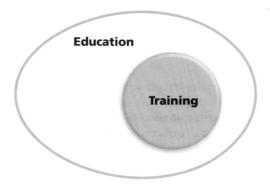

Training, therefore, is *necessary* for PGME but it is not *sufficient* to support or describe the complex process of making professional judgements. For that, we need to turn to the larger term, the white of the egg: education. If a learner's question must be answered with the phrase 'It depends...', then the learner is in an educational environment, rather than a training one, since education concerns itself with the making of complex judgements. Education brings together the underlying rationale of every factor in an equation, to solve problems that are often one-off circumstances, particular to individuals and their needs. It seeks to explore and to balance all of the aspects of all of the circumstances, to arrive at a resolution, which is provisional, and which must be shared with the individuals themselves through a professional conversation. Education examines alternatives and probabilities, bringing to bear all the knowledge, skills and experiences of all the parties in the inquiry. It depends on the matters of fact of training and it uses them to go beyond the general to the particular, to explore possibilities and examine alternatives as they may affect the lived experience of individuals. Where training depends on the results of research for its certainties, education is research in action, balancing probabilities, seeking a synthesis, a provisional, professional judgement which will provide a platform for its next inquiry. What is more, any one professional judgement will reference itself to at least two viewpoints (termed by lawyers 'the margin of appreciation'): a narrow judgement, based entirely on the evidence of the facts of the matter, and a broad judgement, referencing itself to the larger context of the clinical case, to principles and values, and to the larger purposes of individual need.

To this complex interplay between education and training the Greek philosopher Aristotle gave the name 'phronesis', or 'practical wisdom'. It describes the ability to visualise ends, means, and consequences, to relate them to moral lawfulness, and to choose rightly. For this, sufficient experience of particular contexts, as well as of general principles, is required, in order to develop prudent expertise:

> Whereas young people become accomplished in geometry and mathematics, and wise within these limits, prudent young people do not seem to be found. The reason is that prudence is concerned with particulars as well as universals, and particulars become known from experience, but a young person lacks experience, since some length of time is needed to produce it. (*Nicomachaen Ethics* 1142 a)

Underlying Aristotle's formulation, however, was an older philosophical inheritance, which Aristotle had learned from his teacher, Plato. This is the distinction between two kinds of knowledge, 'gnosis' and 'episteme', which stand in relation to each other as education does to training: both to be honoured, both to be recognised as different from each other, but related. It is in the relationship between gnosis and episteme – their distinction and their resolution – that we find the relationship between education and training; between medicine as an art and medicine as a science; and between knowledge and experience.

## Gnosis and Episteme

Raphael's painting, *The School of Athens*, has at its centre the figures of Plato and Aristotle, walking together, deep in conversation. Aristotle, robed in blue, carries a copy of his *Nicomachaen Ethics* in one hand, and with the other gestures outwards, palm down, to the earth below. Plato, robed in red, carries his *Timaeus* in one hand, and with the other points upwards to the heavens. Around them Raphael has painted a pantheon of Greek philosophers and scientists, irrespective of their historical chronology, for his School is neither the Academy founded near Athens by Plato, nor the Lyceum founded by Aristotle on the banks of the Illisus, but a school of the imagination, capturing at once the spirit of the High Renaissance and its inheritances from classical antiquity.

Aristotle, the doctor's son, appeals to the empirical evidence of the material world, the kind of knowledge that, in his *Nicomachaen Ethics*, he termed episteme. This is knowledge of fixed systems, certainties, the incontrovertible facts of the matter, that which is provable by observation. For Aristotle, geometry and mathematics were the exemplars of such fixed systems of knowledge, with the properties of triangles always being deducible from theorems, and vice versa. Other epistemic systems of knowledge include anatomy, astronomy, and botany, while mundane examples of its helpful operation in contemporary everyday life include road-traffic signs, computer manuals, and instructions for filling out a tax return. Episteme arises from the careful observation of the material world, and Aristotle's great contribution to Western thought was the taxonomies that distinguished one thing from another, that separated items and listed them as axioms, as incontrovertible, 'always and only' facts.

Episteme, therefore, is that kind of knowledge that is most amenable to training approaches.

It does not need a rationale, because it is to be learned as axiomatic, as a matter of fact. It requires memorising, not critiquing, and one of the remarkable features of medical education is the sheer quantity of facts which students are required to remember, so that they may know the operation of the human body in all its constituent systems and parts. Training, therefore, provides information about, and instruction in, fixed systems of knowledge. It encompasses the lists and rules which constitute episteme, derived from practice, from the empirical observation of the world about us, as Aristotle's extended hand suggests, and his *Nicomachaen Ethics* elucidates.

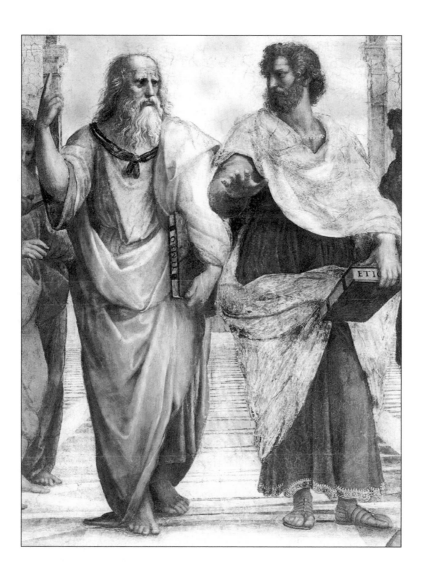

Plato, however, points towards another kind of knowledge: gnosis, the knowledge that is acquired through relationship with the world. Where episteme is concerned with the parts, gnosis is concerned with the whole. In medical terms it is what is meant by a holistic approach: the doctor and patient stand in relationship to each other to explore and co-construct what is best – that is, what is of the highest good – for that individual, in those circumstances, with the options available. Crucially, gnosis arises from the exploration of relationality, using intuition and seeking insight into the world of others, and so it is created in a specific context. This complex and deeply personal exploration constitutes the process of education, and explains why Peters describes education as a conversation: because it must be a shared exploration, whether as a discussion between individuals or as the interior dialogue between an individual and their world, that produces art, literature, music, and philosophy. Ultimately, the purpose of the conversation is to experience and elucidate qualitative understandings, the ethical and aesthetic values that make up the rich, textured quality of life: what constitutes right action, what is the good, the true, the beautiful.

It is in his *Timaeus* that Plato makes his clearest statements about gnosis and its purpose, which is not simply to provide spiritual enlightenment for the individual, but to bring about a morally lawful way of life for the good of all, in a world which is 'a single, visible living being, containing within itself all living beings of the same natural order' (*Timaeus* §30). However, in the seventh letter of his *Epistles*, Plato is also clear that this cannot be achieved through rote learning, but manifests itself as the result of a long, shared inquiry between teacher and learner:

> This knowledge is not something that can be put into words like other sciences; but after long-continued intercourse between teacher and pupil, in joint pursuit of the subject, suddenly, like light flashing forth when a fire is kindled, it is born in the soul and straightway nourishes itself (*Epistles* §341 c).

To produce its 'eureka' moments, its epiphanies of insight, gnosis requires an imaginative understanding as well as a simply factual one: Fleming has to see beyond the dirty petri dishes into the imaginative potential of the penicillin bacterium; or, as Jim Watson described his breakthrough in DNA (1970, 148-9, 163):

> I no sooner got to the office and began explaining my scheme than the American crystallographer Jerry Donohue protested that the idea would not work. The tautomeric forms I had copied out of Davidson's book were, in Jerry's opinion, incorrectly assigned. My immediate retort that several other texts also pictured guanine and thymine in the enol form cut no ice with Jerry. Happily, he let out that for years organic chemists had been arbitrarily favouring particular tautomeric forms over their alternatives on only the flimsiest of grounds. The guanine picture I was thrusting towards his face was almost certainly bogus. All his chemical intuition told him that it would occur in the keto form. He was just as sure that thymine was also wrongly assigned an enol configuration. Again he strongly favoured the keto alternative...

> The unforeseen dividend of having Jerry share an office with Francis, Peter and me, though obvious to all, was not spoken about. If he had not been with us in Cambridge, I might still have been pumping for a like-with-like structure… But for Jerry, only Pauling would have been likely to make the right choice and stick by its consequences.

In human terms, this reaching for understanding through imaginative relationality is called compassion: the act of seeing oneself in the other person, and wishing to treat them as one would wish to be treated by them. This happens in reality, not in the abstract, and the relationship has to be sought anew each time, just as a painting, or a piece of music, or a poem, must be understood again each time it is seen or heard or read. What is sought is a connection with eternal moral values, called 'Forms' by Plato, which will illuminate (literally, 'light up') our understanding of the 'facts' – the pigment on canvas, the vibrations from strings, the ink on paper – that are so carefully delineated by episteme. Gnosis is a reverberant, qualitative knowledge, which seeks to make facts transparent to the possibilities that lie beyond them, the potentials into which they may combine, and the moral lawfulness that attends those alternatives.

Raphael has painted Plato's light, mobile figure as a direct link between the material world, in which he stands barefoot, and the world of imaginative insight, to which his raised hand points, and has made a circle of continuity to the easily carried *Timaeus*, where Plato describes the relationship between eternal values and lived experience. By contrast, the figure of Aristotle seems static, foreshortened to stillness by his outreaching hand, and with his progress impeded by the weighty *Nicomachaen Ethics* resting clumsily on his thigh, suggesting that episteme without gnosis is, in the end, more of a hindrance than a help. However, Raphael has linked the two together, overlapping them, so that Plato's walk, and his glance beyond Aristotle, moves the younger philosopher along with him, suggesting, perhaps, the moral obligation of the educator to help the learner to proceed: a practical example of an imaginative, compassionate sharing of worlds.

## Whole and Part

As Tarnas (1991, 68-72) points out, taken together Aristotle and Plato represent an 'elegant balance and tension between empirical analysis and spiritual intuition' with an 'accompanying creative tension and complexity,' which provided Western philosophy with 'a dual legacy' that has been fundamental and enduring. Crucially, it reveals a relationship between a whole and a part, in which a larger term contains a smaller one, and makes meaning of it. Education, with its demand for an ethically based rationale and its provisional, exploratory conversations, contains training, with its information, tips, and facts, just as gnosis contains episteme.

The relationship between the part and the whole, the inevitable fragmentation of our experience in order to survive physically in the world, together with the overwhelming need to experience its wholeness, in order to find value in our lives, both builds on, and pre-dates, classical Greek thought. It is exemplified by the work of two contemporary philosophers, David Bohm and Jules Cashford. Bohm's *Wholeness and the Implicate Order* develops a rational and scientific theory, based on quantum physics, which treats the totality of existence, including matter and consciousness, as an unbroken whole. He comments:

> It is instructive to consider that the word 'health' in English is based on an Anglo-Saxon word 'hale' meaning 'whole': that is, to be healthy is to be whole, which is, I think, roughly the equivalent of the Hebrew 'shalem'. Likewise, the English 'holy' is based on the same root as 'whole'. All of this indicates that man has sensed always that wholeness or integrity is an absolute necessity to make life worth living. Yet, over the ages, he has generally lived in fragmentation (Bohm 1980, 3).

This fragmentation, Bohm (1980, 8) suggests, arises out of individuals' need to separate off pieces of experience in order to understand them, and he recognises that this has produced remarkable insights:

> Consider, for example, the atomic theory, which was first proposed by Democritus more than 2,000 years ago. In essence, this theory leads us to look at the world as constituted of atoms, moving in the void. The ever-changing forms and characteristics of large-scale objects are now seen as the results of changing arrangements of the moving atoms. Evidently, this view was, in certain ways, an important mode of realization of wholeness, for it enabled men to understand the enormous variety of the whole world in terms of the movement of one single set of basic constituents, through a single void that permeates the whole of existence. Nevertheless, as the atomic theory developed, it ultimately became a major support for a fragmentary approach to reality. For it ceased to be regarded as an insight, a way of looking, and men regarded instead as an absolute truth the notion that the whole of reality is actually constituted of nothing but 'atomic building blocks', all working together more or less mechanically.

Quantum theory, of course, challenged such a view, revealing that light is both a particle and a wave, and thereby suggesting that a new set of relationships remained to be discovered. However, as Bohm (1980, 8) points out, what is required is not a new, more integrated way of thinking, but a fundamental recognition that ideas of fragmentation and integration are themselves illusory:

> What should be said is that wholeness is what is real, and that fragmentation is the response of this whole to man's action, guided by illusory perception, which is shaped by fragmentary thought… So what is needed is for man to give attention to his habit of fragmentary thought, to be aware of it, and thus bring it to an end… What is called for is not an *integration* of thought, or a kind of imposed unity, for any such imposed point of view would itself be merely another fragment. Rather, all our different ways of thinking

are to be considered as different ways of looking at the one reality…The whole object is not perceived in any one view, but, rather, it is grasped only *implicitly* as that single reality which is shown in all these views.

Bohm's vision of wholeness is, of course, Plato's vision of 'the One', described in *Timaeus*, where Plato also begins the fragmentation process by breaking down the implicate order into four elements of fire, water, air, and earth, in order to describe and understand their combination in people and their implications for medical care. Crucially, knowledge gained from empirical observation and knowledge gained through relationships are interdependent: in Kant's famous formulation, 'Thoughts without concepts are empty… intuitions without concepts are blind' (*Critique of Pure Reason*, A51).

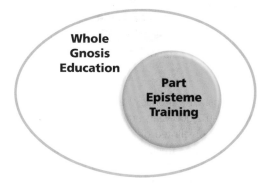

## Zoe and Bios

Taken together, however, gnosis and episteme reveal a larger relationship which, in contemporary scientific terms, Bohm calls 'the implicate order', and for which Jules Cashford employs the classical Greek terms 'zoe' and 'bios'. Tracing the evolution of the implicate order from the sensibility evidenced by Palaeolithic art to the contemporary European mind, Cashford says:

> This essential distinction between the whole and the part was later formulated in the Greek language by the two different Greek words for life, zoe and bios, as the embodiment of two dimensions co-existing in life. *Zoe* is eternal and infinite life; *bios* is the living and dying manifestation of this eternal world in time. The Classical scholar Carl Kerenyi explains: 'Zoe is the thread upon which every individual *bios* is strung like a bead, and which, in contrast to bios, can be conceived of only as endless' – as 'infinite life' (Baring and Cashford 1991, 148).

The awareness that 'life in time' is held within 'life in eternity' reveals another relationship – that between the finite, like people, and the infinite, such as the universe. This means that people belong to the world, rather than the world belonging to people, an understanding that is fundamental to contemporary concerns about ecology and conservation. Suddenly, a vision of the world that seemed new and marginal, is revealed as a fundamental part of human consciousness. Each is lived through the other, encouraging a constant exploration of relationships, that is at once imaginative and practical. It is here, finally, in the implicit moral order, that principles and practice catalyse each other into new knowledge, requiring us to determine where we stand in relationship to everyone and everything: this is education.

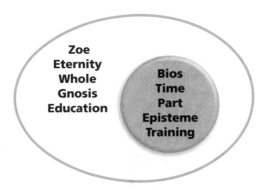

## Getting It Wrong

An adequate rationale for education, then, lies in a series of relationships, rightly held: the relationship between principles and practice; between education and training; between gnosis and episteme; and between zoe and bios, as the infinite and the finite, eternity and time, the whole and the part. Education requires an imaginative exploration of these relationships by the individual, an exploration which is fundamentally a felt, ethical inquiry. At its moral centre is what Huxley (1946, 2) calls 'the perennial philosophy', the principle of compassion, which he traces through world religions. This principle is held in common by all spiritual paths, and it requires us to recognise ourselves in others, and thus to treat others as we would wish to be treated ourselves. Huxley refers us to the Sanskrit formula, *tat tvam asi* ('That art thou'). A secular expression of this spiritual value is provided by Kant, as the 'Categorical Imperative', that is, as an absolute principle for the conduct of human affairs (*Groundwork of the Metaphysics of Morals*, 4:421). The Categorical Imperative has three requirements: that we should act as though our action was a universal law, that will affect us as well as others; that we treat all of humanity, including ourselves, as ends in their own right, not as means to an end; and that we should act as though all our actions will bring into being a world of ends. It is these principles that lie behind both the playground cry of 'It's not fair!' and the medical insider's gold-standard for clinical care, 'Would you let this person attend a member of your family?' Both circumstances make a fundamental appeal to individual compassion and to the implicit moral order, and both express felt, lived experience of relationship.

But what about when things go wrong, when the learner is devastated, or the patient harmed? This question has been a source of ethical concern from the earliest recorded times, as we can learn from the first story that we have written down, the Mesopotamian *Epic of Gilgamesh*. There, the hero, Gilgamesh, victorious King of Uruk, decides to kill the lord of the forest, Humbaba:

He said to his servant Enkidu, 'I have not established my name stamped on brick as my destiny decreed; therefore I will go to the country where the cedar is felled, I will set up my name in the place where the names of famous men are written'… 'We will go to the forest and destroy the evil, for in the forest lives Humbaba whose name is "Hugeness", a ferocious giant'… 'Then if I fall I leave behind me a name that endures: men will say, "Gilgamesh has fallen in fight with ferocious Humbaba." Long after the child has been born in my house, they will say it and remember' (Sandars 1960, 68-9).

Gilgamesh ignores his faithful companion, Enkidu, who implores: 'Do not abuse this power, deal justly.' Enkidu himself is drawn into the desire for victory at all costs, so that when Humbaba piteously appeals to Gilgamesh for compassion, it is denied him, and he is slain. There is a moment when one appeals to the compassion of the other, asking as a universal principle of mercy, 'Should not the snared bird return to its nest, and the captive man return to his mother's arms?' (Sandars 1960, 81). However, Humbaba has become a means to the end of Gilgamesh's personal glory, and so must be destroyed.

Crucially, it is not just that Gilgamesh and Enkidu breach the implicit moral order that advocates compassion, but that they break it intentionally and knowingly, and it is precisely this that the writer was at pains to point out 4,000 years ago. They thus incur *moral guilt*, that is, the personal guilt arising from the deliberate intention to do harm, and the rest of the epic deals with Gilgamesh's sense of desolation arising from his moral guilt, and the terrible journey he undertakes to try to expiate it.

This is quite different from setting out with good intentions and carefulness, yet somehow failing because of circumstances beyond your control. To that experience the Greeks (Kitto 1951, 170) gave the name 'hamartia', with the image of an arrow missing the mark. The archer aims attentively at the centre of the target, but the arrow is taken astray by external factors, so that it misses the mark. As the metaphor indicates, such a stray arrow may be no less deadly than an aimed one, but the intention is not to do harm and thus the ethical bond is honoured. Hamartia gives rise to *tragic guilt*, which does not belong to the actor but to the way of the world and, indeed, may not be owned by the actor. Rather, it must be located within what the Greeks called 'Ananke', implacable fate, necessity, serving as a reminder to the actor that some things are beyond their control. Circumstances such as these, above all, delineate the interplay between practice and principle, and the need to live within, rather than live against, the complexities of an imperfect world.

# Vulnerability

KSS Education Department's approach, therefore, is to take a set of ethical principles directly into practice, into real-life, complex, problematic clinical settings, with the expectation that those principles will be refined and exemplified by practice. The vision is of education as a whole, an interweaving of principles and practice, gnosis and episteme, a reconciliation of the different kinds of knowledge called by Ryle (1949, 25-61) 'knowing that' and 'knowing how'. The quality that education, in this fuller sense, provides for individuals is typified by Peters (1966, 30) as 'transformation', since 'education implies that a man's outlook is transformed by what he knows', and it is to be achieved through 'conversation':

> The question is whether explicit learning situations are sufficient to bring about this integrated outlook. The classical way of ensuring this, surely, has been not courses but conversation. Conversation is not structured like a discussion group in terms of one form of thought, or towards the solution of a problem. In a conversation, lecturing to others is bad form; so is using the remarks of others as springboards for self-display. The point is to create a common world to which all bring their distinctive contributions.

The 'distinctive contribution' which KSS ADEs bring to professional conversations is their expertise in education, which will usually have been their lifelong vocation, just as medicine has been the lifelong vocation of the doctors with whom they work. This suggests vulnerability on both sides. ADEs are guests in the world of medicine, seeking to make sense of an environment which is foreign to them, while focusing on educational processes with which they have long and intimate acquaintance. Similarly, clinicians are opening up their practice to scrutiny by experts whose knowledge of education is as great as their own knowledge of their clinical specialty. Both have as their shared focus the best interests of the learner and a recognition that good teaching produces good patient care. They must explore each other's worlds, share understandings, and develop agreements about what constitutes acceptable practice, in a particular place, at a particular time, and under particular circumstances. These two experts must negotiate between them what Benhabib (1992, 25) calls 'the transfer of the power and prerogative of judgement', so that each empowers the other to discuss their different, temporarily shared, areas of professional practice. These discussions take place in the highly politicised contexts of PGME, and as Benhabib (1992, 25) points out, 'judgement, as a social process of appropriating and exercising knowledge, can become a political question'. Ultimately, however, the professional conversation about education in clinical settings is structured by a shared ethical concern, which differentiates it from political questions:

> Moral judgement differs from these other domains in one crucial respect: the exercise of moral judgement is pervasive and unavoidable; in fact, this exercise is coextensive with relations of social interaction in the lifeworld in general. Moral judgement is what we 'always already' exercise in virtue of our being immersed in a network of human relationships that constitute our life together (Benhabib 1992, 25).

The real, shared concern of educationists and clinicians, therefore, is that their professional judgements should be morally lawful, not that they should be politically appropriate. Like Gilgamesh and Enkidu, they face moral choices at each turn of their professional conversation. In particular, they are acutely aware that people – their learners and their patients respectively – may not be treated as means to an end, for to do so would be to deny their autonomy, their freedom to choose, and thus their moral agency. As Barfield (1953,

121) points out, the word 'heretic' is derived from the Greek 'hairetikos', 'able to choose', and in that sense doctors and teachers, and patients and learners, are all necessary heretics, if the practice of medicine and education is to be ethical.

There is, therefore, a necessary sense of uncertainty and displacement in the practice of education in clinical settings, which might be considered as a particular form of consciousness, called by Braidotti (1994, 25) a 'nomadic consciousness':

> Nomadic consciousness is akin to what Foucault called countermemory; it is a form of resisting assimilation or homolgation into dominant ways of representing the self… The nomadic style is about transitions and passages without predetermined destinations or lost homelands. The nomad's relationship to the earth is one of transitory attachment and cyclical frequentation; the antithesis of the farmer, the nomad gathers, reaps, and exchanges but does not exploit.

The professional conversation takes place in the zone of contact between education and medicine, a liminal area, the 'third space', an essentially moral dimension that is discussed by Pam Shaw in Chapter 3 and Rachel Robinson in Chapter 4 of this book. In marrying practice with principles it is a discussion that is at once tentative, provisional and uncertain, and assured, acute and precise. It has the qualities that the novelist Thomas Mann ascribed to 'lunar syntax', and which his faithful correspondent, the mythologist Karl Kerenyi, termed 'Hermetic'. For Mann (1933, 77-8), 'things look differently under the moon and under the sun, and it might be the clearness of the moon which would appeal to the spirit as the truer clarity', so that an individual's personal narrative necessarily 'opened at the back, as it were, and overflowed into spheres external to his own individuality both in space and in time', not least because 'the conception of individuality belongs after all to the same category of conceptions as that of unity and entirety, the whole and the all.' In Mann's capacity for moving in this proximal zone, where individual and eternal realities intercalate, Kerenyi (1975, 6-7) found 'an embodiment of that Hermetic spirit…He moved in this realm of human existence, this border area between life and death, as the Greeks believed their god Hermes did. The spiritual reality of the god Hermes, the basis of the faith he once inspired, involved a capability that, after all, also corresponds to an exceptional capacity of the mind: to be at home even in that realm.'

It is the role of the educationist to bring the moral unconscious into consciousness, to support the learner in bringing that which they have 'always already' known, the implicate order, into their professional practice. This is the 'transformation' to which Peters refers. It is the role of the clinician to be at home in the 'border area between life and death' and to initiate their learners into that exceptional practice. This is the fundamental transformation of human existence. Between these two transformative practices and seeking to capture them, both allusively and exactly, lie the professional conversations, accounts of 'how it is' and 'how it might be' that are a complex synthesis of externally derived knowledge, mediated through personal experience – stories that change, perhaps, in the re-telling, and in their changes move on both the teller and their auditor.

The remainder of this book is devoted to KSS Education Department's reflections on some of these 'conversations from the field'.

# References

Aristotle. 1976. *Ethics*. Translated by J.A.K. Thomson, revised by Hugh Tredennick and edited by Betty Radice. London, Penguin.

Barfield, O. 1953. *History in English Words*. London: Faber and Faber.

Baring A. & J. Cashford. 1991. *The Myth of the Goddess: Evolution of an Image*. London: Viking.

Barrow R. & R. Woods. 1988. *An Introduction to the Philosophy of Education*. London: Routledge.

Benhabib, S. 1992. *Situating the Self: Gender, Community and Postmodernism in Contemporary Ethics*. Cambridge: Polity Press.

Bohm, D. 1980. *Wholeness and the Implicate Order*. London: Routledge.

Braidotti, R. 1994. *Nomadic Subjects: Embodiment and Sexual Difference in Contemporary Feminist theory*. New York: Columbia University Press.

de Cossart L. & D. Fish. 2005. *Cultivating a Thinking Surgeon*. Shrewsbury: tfm Publishing.

Eraut, M. 1994. *Developing Professional Knowledge and Competence*. London: Falmer Press.

Huxley, A. 1946. *The Perennial Philosophy*. London: Chatto & Windus.

Kant, I. 1996. Groundwork of the Metaphysic of Morals (1785). In *Practical Philosophy*. Translated and edited by Mary J. Gregor. Cambridge: CUP.

Kant, I. 1998. *Critique of Pure Reason*. Translated and edited by Paul Guyer. Cambridge: CUP.

Kerenyi, K. 1975. *Mythology and Humanism: the Correspondence of Thomas Mann and Karl Kerenyi*. Translated by Alexander Gelley. London: Cornell University Press.

Kitto, H. D. F. 1951. *The Greeks*. Harmondsworth: Penguin.

Mann, T. 1999. *Joseph and His Brothers*. Translated by H. T. Lowe-Porter. London: Vintage.

Oakeshott, M. 1962. *Rationalism in Politics: And other Essays*. London: Methuen.

Peters, R. S. 1966. *Ethics and Education*. London: Allen & Unwin.

Peters, R. S. 1967. What is an Educational Process? *The Concept of Education*. London: Routledge and Kegan Paul.

Plato. 1962. *Epistles*. Translated by Glenn R. Morrow. New York: Bobbs-Merrill.

Plato. 1971. Timaeus. *Timaeus and Critias*. Translated by Desmond Lee and edited by Betty Radice. London: Penguin.

Playdon Z. J. & D. Goodsman.1997. Education or Training: Medicine's Learning Agenda. *British Medical Journal* 314. 29 March 1997. 983-4.

Ryle, G. 1949. *The Concept of Mind*. London:Hutchinson.

Sandars, N. 1960. *The Epic of Gilgamesh*. Harmondsworth: Penguin Books.

Stone, E. 1992. *Quality Teaching: a Sample of Cases*. London: Routledge.

Tarnas, R. 1991. *The Passion of the Western Mind*. New York: Ballantine Books.

Watson, J. D. 1970. *The Double Helix*. London: Penguin.

# Faculty and Governance: Not Lost in Translation but Held in Transition

## Context

In recent years I have become particularly interested in how organisations work, and how change within them can be managed well. As Deputy Head of Education at Kent, Surrey and Sussex Postgraduate Medical Deanery [KSS], I have become increasingly aware that the Education Department takes up a 'boundary' position in relation to the rest of the organisation. Part of the challenge of inhabiting the position of Assistant Dean Education [ADE] within KSS's predominantly clinical and workforce-oriented organisation is knowing how to take up the role with authority, assurance and, most importantly, with legitimacy. I was struck by Wenger's (1998, 109) comments that partnership within and between communities of practice (in this context, between the Education Department and the wider organisational system of KSS) require a brokering function:

> The job of brokering is complex. It involves processes of translation, coordination, and alignment between perspectives. It requires enough legitimacy to influence the development of a practice, mobilize attention and address conflicting interests. It also requires the ability to link practices by facilitating transactions between them and to cause learning by introducing into a practice elements of another.

Given Wenger's comments, I am interested not only in the nature of the legitimacy required by non-medical, senior academic ADEs to take up their role, but also in the contributions which psychoanalytic and systemic thinking can bring to the ways in which organisations function well or poorly. I am interested in issues both 'above the surface' and 'below the surface' within organisations. I am also interested in the idea of creating a 'third space' within organisations, where ideas that are on the periphery of an organisation's vision can be slowly brought into view, and considered in a way which goes beyond the binary opposition of 'the doer and the done to' (Benjamin 2004, 5). The third space, in this context, is primarily based on relationships and partnership between stakeholders, and is a locus in which authority must be negotiated.

As I see it, this third space would be a co-created location for thinking about, and enacting, organisational change. In my work at KSS, I have sought to support this type of change through a 'process consultancy' approach (Schein 1988; 1990), that is, an approach where the *process* of addressing an issue is as important as the issue itself.

Recently we have seen a period of unprecedented, turbulent, and rapid change within postgraduate medical education [PGME]. Current initiatives include the introduction of mandated entitlement curricula for Foundation Programme [Foundation] and specialty PGME, and the introduction of specialty 'run-through' programmes. Local Education Providers [LEPs] manage, monitor, and are accountable for the educational opportunities they offer to postgraduate doctors. In this context PGME has become a political locus of educational governance, centralised within the General Medical Council [GMC]. In this new structure, the GMC is responsible for quality assurance; Postgraduate Medical Deaneries [Deaneries] are responsible for quality management; and LEPs are responsible for quality control. This structure represents a more stringent, formalised, top-down, educational governance structure for PGME than has existed hitherto.

## Purposes

KSS Education Department responded to these educational governance initiatives by creating a change-management process that reflected our participative and democratic ethos. This work built on the processes used in our system of Contract Review, which we have developed iteratively, in collaboration with our LEPs, over a period of eighteen years. Through the Contract Review process, each LEP is visited annually by a KSS team, led by an ADE, in order to review progress and support local development. Our aim, therefore, was to work with colleagues in LEPs who were involved in educational governance at differing levels of engagement and responsibility, to collaborate in devising and developing new systems, which would function well, and retain a sound educational focus. We wanted to ensure that, through the participation of those closely involved in PGME, these education governance systems would be viable, useful, and appropriate, rather than a layer of centrally imposed bureaucracy.

My account of the way we achieved our purposes will look briefly at the impact of the European Working Time Regulations [EWTR], and at the emergence of National Curriculum Frameworks [NCFs] for specialty PGME. Then, I will consider the significance of PGME's location within a loosely coupled authority structure, that is, one which has high autonomy relative to the larger system in which it sits. From here, I shall outline an educational change process within KSS, defining this as one of process consultancy, working towards a devolved and decentralised model of LEP authority and accountability, and seeking to support 'earned autonomy' at LEP level. My account will highlight the importance of having established transitional 'holding structures' while LEPs moved to locally owned educational governance and quality control. In this context, I shall offer the work of Krantz (2001) as a useful lens for considering change management. While discussing the dilemmas of organisational change, Krantz proposes a basic framework, which takes account of contributory factors leading to what he calls 'primitive' or 'sophisticated' change. A 'primitive change', as defined by Krantz, is one in which there is either an 'idealised even utopian conception', or, alternatively 'rampant cynicism'. By contrast, in the 'sophisticated' stance, he suggests, 'people are able to adopt a hopeful attitude towards the future, tempered by an appreciation of the challenges involved in achieving new approaches' (Krantz 2001, 141).

Throughout my account, I will present process consultancy as an apposite, underpinning model of change agency. This view is illustrated by three brief, inter-related case studies of process consultancy in practice. These show how we established 'holding structures' that supported each LEP's emergent autonomy, providing a process analogous to Krantz's 'sophisticated' stance towards change management.

## Change within a Networked World

Over the past decade, change has affected PGME at every level, and at a frantic pace. Competing, and sometimes incompatible, innovations have been implemented within relatively short time frames, often involving a range of stakeholders with differing agendas. PGME is not alone in experiencing intrusion (and sometimes surveillance) by increasingly centralised government agencies; an erosion of public trust in professional institutions such as schools, universities, and the NHS, has led to a general demand for increased public accountability, regulation, and performance management. Within these professions there has been a move towards an audit culture, where professional judgement and self-regulation are replaced by an accountability framework, which is primarily instrumental and technocratic in its focus. Competency frameworks are ubiquitous in these technocratic approaches, and have recently been introduced in PGME, although they are highly problematic in educational environments. The alternative, of course, is to develop accountability frameworks based on the professional values inherent in social practices, such as medicine (MacIntyre 1981).

## Organisational Change

Broader contemporary changes and pressures have also influenced the ways in which organisations function and are structured. These include, for instance, the increasing importance of information technology, and increasing recognition of multiple organisational stakeholders. This has led to the emergence of what Cooper and Dartington (2004, 142) have described as a 'vanishing organisation'. They suggest that, in the 'vanishing organisation', a more traditional, hierarchically held structure is giving way to one which is more horizontal, thus affording opportunities for less centralised responses to stakeholders, and also for creativity, devolved local autonomy, networking, and relationality. The LEPs with whom we work frequently occupy both positions at the same time. They are still quite traditional, hierarchically, and thus are vertically structured, and yet they also have to recognise and respond to different stakeholder agendas, which can lead to a more horizontal, devolved structure, with a focus on partnership working.

PGME is not unaffected by these changes. Within PGME, there are often competing and potentially incompatible demands, as in the concurrent emergence of NCFs and EWTR. EWTR limit the amount of time postgraduate doctors can spend in the workplace, while NCFs set out a work-based curriculum, which may require more time for completion by specific individuals than EWTR allows. Eraut (2008) provides an apposite illustration of external pressures on surgical training. He suggests that these are: EWTR, increasing public expectations for accountability and transparency, and new working practices and service delivery. He explains:

> [given] shift working for both trainers and trainees in several branches of
> medicine . . . the EWTD will reach its final figure of 48 hrs per week in 2009
> . . . this has significantly reduced the time that trainees can spend in the
> formal and informal learning environments. This situation has been further
> exacerbated by the growth of subspecialties . . . the combination of both
> these factors has led to the dissolution of the firm structure (Eraut 2008, 1).

Continuing concern about the incompatibility of the requirements of EWTR and NCFs has led recently to a Modernising Medical Careers [MMC] publication, dealing specifically with managing the reduction of hours for PGME. *MMC Programme Board Task and Finish Group on Quality: Maintaining Quality of Training in a Reduced Training Opportunity Environment* recommends:

> A planning group must be established in each Local Education Provider [LEP]
> to consider innovative approaches to maintaining quality of training in the
> light of reduced training opportunities (MMC 2009, 4).

The 'firm structure', to which Eraut refers, is the medical team in a hospital specialty, headed by a consultant, staffed by postgraduate doctors, and known traditionally as a 'Firm' (Moss 1995). There is a significant possibility that the status of the professional judgement of clinicians as teachers may be diminished as a consequence of the dissolution of the 'firm structure', which held PGME within an informal 'community of practice' (Wenger 1998). Further, there are related concerns that GMC's centralisation of educational governance, and the new, centralised NCFs may lead to deprofessionalisation, particularly of clinicians as teachers. Interestingly, a recent keynote speech to the Association for Medical Education Europe [AMEE], referred to the volume of 'political imperatives which impact on PGME, which produces a crowded arena in which the voice of practising clinicians and the profession as a whole can be lost' (Grant 2009).

From this volatile context emerge several issues that impact on the educational integrity of PGME. KSS and its LEPs are required to engage with NCFs within the context of EWTR's reduction in opportunities for teaching and learning PGME, at a time of organisational restructuring.

## Mandated Entitlement Specialty Curricula: a Slow Walk to Professional Freedom?

GMC, in collaboration with MMC and the medical Royal Colleges [Royal Colleges], has agreed what are *de facto* mandated entitlement NCFs for postgraduate doctors across all specialties. Almost inevitably, this development has produced a Janus-faced position. On the one hand, it offers a most welcome learner entitlement, and a requirement for curriculum specificity. Mandated NCFs safeguard both learner and teacher by demanding clarity about the roles, responsibilities, and expectations of all those involved in curriculum implementation. This includes consultant teachers, postgraduate doctors, and programme leaders, as well as Medical Education Managers [MEMs], and administrators, whose support is crucial to the effective running of the programmes. Further, such curricula need to be held within KSS and local educational governance structures to ensure their integrity. On the other hand, however, the centralisation of curricula may lead to a sense of deprofessionalisation. Curriculum development, regulation, and accountability may be perceived as solely the province of central authorities, rather than as an area benefiting from local professional judgement, tacit knowledge, and 'know-how'.

The challenge, as we saw it as an Education Department, was to attend to the issues raised by NCFs, EWTR, and new structures for educational governance, but to do so in ways which supported both learner entitlement, and the professional integrity of consultants as teachers. Therefore, we adopted a process consultancy model, intending to provide holding frames, in which professional judgement and deliberation could flourish, while at the same time offering an educationally sound governance structure, which could complement that of the GMC. As educationists with backgrounds in Higher Education Institutions [HEIs], we had experience of the holding structures usual in mainstream university practice, such as Academic Boards, and Faculty Groups. This experience provided both a legitimacy, and a template for establishing such holding frameworks in PGME. Furthermore, the understandings and concerns brought to the table by clinicians involved locally in PGME, ensured a genuine negotiation, and sharing of authority, as we grappled with the new requirements.

## PGME within a Loosely Coupled Structure

Organisationally, PGME sits within a 'loosely coupled' structure, in so far as education for postgraduate doctors is work-based, and devolved to LEPs. Hirschhorn (1997, 1) has defined a loosely coupled structure as one:

in which individual elements have high autonomy relative to the larger system that they are in, often having a federated character. In loosely coupled systems, the forces for integration . . . for worrying about the whole, its identity, its integrity and its future . . . are often weak compared to the forces for specialization. Central authority is derived as much from the members versus the member elements receiving delegated authority from above.

There is, of course, a formal Education Contract between KSS and each of its LEPs. But PGME is also nested within a complex context of relationships between different LEPs. So, as well as individual contractual relationships, there is also something close to a federated relationship between KSS and its LEPs, which depends on negotiated autonomy and partnership.

## Educational Approaches and Models of Change

The models of change management most influential on the Education Department's approach to supporting PGME 'in transition' were those of process consultancy and action research. Process consultancy, as described by Schein (1988; 1990), is less concerned with the content of a problem, and more with the process by which an individual, group, or organisation identifies and solves a problem. Thus, we sought to attend to issues current in PGME in a way which would make maximum use of local professional deliberation and judgement, and which would support local autonomy and the professional judgement of consultants as teachers. Intrinsic to the change process, therefore, was the idea of *partnership in practice*. We sought to promote a change model that was based on partnership between KSS Education Department, our LEPs, their Directors of Medical Education [DMEs], and their MEMs and their Educational Supervisors.

Krantz (2001, 152) offers a most useful lens for thinking about the inherent difficulties and challenges of change agency within a loosely coupled system such as PGME. He suggests that organisational change frequently leads to anxiety, and that this in itself needs to be attended to. He makes a useful distinction between 'sophisticated' and 'primitive' models of change agency, and suggests that organisations need support when they move through inevitable transitional phases, as they seek to accommodate change. He characterises *primitive* change as that which, for example, includes innovation overload caused by too much change within too short a time frame, or change which lacks appropriate structures to contain the change process. Krantz further suggests that *sophisticated* change requires:

> genuine investment in structures designed to contain and address issues pertaining to the change process; realistic assessment of the time required to effect significant change; clarity about how the change effort represents continuity as well as discontinuity; toleration of learning from inevitable mistakes . . . articulation of a plausible and compelling picture of the future that is commonly shared and understood (2001, 152).

With this in mind, and with a wish to provide authoritative containing structures within the loosely coupled structure of PGME, we set about a change process to support educational governance, and curricula entitlement. We described this process to ourselves as one that was 'not lost in translation but held in transition'. The Education Department's strategy was to provide a variety of 'holding frameworks' to support educational governance. These are outlined in some detail below. We have a history of very good partnership working with LEPs, and we believed that this experience, combined with our recognition of KSS's loosely coupled, federated relationship with its LEPs, could be built on to create a model of educational governance that would be sensitive and responsive to local contexts, while supporting local professional educational judgement, and professional autonomy.

## How This Worked in Practice: Three Brief Case Studies

Three short case studies follow, which exemplify the Education Department's progress towards a model of 'sophisticated' change agency. This involved three key initiatives: the introduction of the concept of Local Faculty Groups [LFGs]; the development of a KSS educational governance structure, the *Graduate Education and Assessment Regulations* [GEAR 2010]; and the development of a cadre of senior higher-education professionals, with a remit specifically to support the development of LFGs. Each of the three initiatives was underpinned by our working in partnership with a range of key stakeholders, from KSS, Royal Colleges, and LEPs. All three initiatives were brought about through change management, which was based on process consultancy. In turn, our process consultancy engaged us in lateral relationships; required us to create 'holding' structures; called upon the continuing support of professional 'know-how'; and supported a move to locally devolved autonomy. Each of the three initiatives, and each of the aspects of our process consultancy functioned in slightly different ways to stabilise the turbulent world of PGME, but all of them were conceptualised as a means of facilitating LEP-earned autonomy, and as support for the professional judgement of clinicians working in KSS LEPs.

## *Setting Up Local Faculties for Foundation*

An initial impetus for change was the introduction of Foundation for postgraduate doctors in 2005. KSS Education Department took a process-consultancy approach to Foundation curriculum development, and established what we then called 'working parties' within each LEP, to create a local programme that fulfilled national requirements. Typically, these local working parties comprised Foundation Directors, Educational Supervisors, MEMs, and Information and Technology [IT] colleagues. An ADE worked in partnership with them, as part of a community of practice, on local Foundation curriculum development, building on existing best practice. The approach used by ADEs was that of an ongoing 'professional conversation' about existing best practice, both clinical and educational, and how that might be developed locally for Foundation to meet the new requirements.

It soon became evident that there needed to be an organising principle or *holding framework* for this work. We decided that the development of a Local Foundation Handbook for both postgraduate doctors and Educational Supervisors would provide a necessary focus or organising principle. As these working parties progressed, it was clear that, in each LEP, there was developing a local collegiate partnership, which afforded a significant critical mass of clinicians and managers working together on PGME. The working parties provided a forum where existing best practice in education and management could be both discussed and creatively shaped. As an Education Department we felt that this was a crucial and fundamental source of local professional 'know-how' and expertise, which needed to be preserved, and that, rather than disbanding the working parties after six months of work, they needed to be maintained and supported. Pragmatically, we saw this as particularly important in relation to securing the requirements of the new Foundation curriculum to meet KSS's performance targets. However, we also saw that maintaining the working parties as a critical mass of clinicians and managers offered the potential for a robust framework for local educational governance, akin to the very well-established practices in university faculties. This gave rise to re-framing, and naming the workshop group in each LEP as a 'Foundation Local Faculty Group'. The format we developed in this way is now part of recent national best practice for Foundation, so that the *UK Foundation Programme Curriculum* (2010, 48) currently states:

> Therefore the local Foundation Programme training director / tutor should ensure that there is a local faculty responsible for forming a balanced judgement of a doctor's performance, supported by the assessment results.

Our original concept of a KSS LFG was that it should comprise a Foundation Chair, an Educational Supervisor, a MEM and postgraduate doctors. It was mandated to meet three times a year, track postgraduate doctor progression in a confidential section of the meeting, and ensure postgraduate doctor representation and feedback. Foundation LFGs were seen as a means of devolving autonomy and responsibility within each LEP.

## *Specialty LFGs and Local Academic Boards*

At the point at which NCFs were being introduced, the LFG concept was extended beyond Foundation to create LFGs for specialty PGME in every KSS LEP. It was evident, however, that there were too many specialty LFGs in each LEP for them to be effective units of management for the DME. An integrating and overarching unit of management was called for. This was achieved in two complementary ways: the introduction of GEAR, and the concept and practice of a Local Academic Board [LAB]. In GEAR we wrote and articulated a set of governing principles for LFGs and LABs. This regulatory framework again mirrored HEI practices, in so far as each HEI in the UK has an academic board, which oversees the delivery of postgraduate courses within its remit. Each HEI also has a statement of learner entitlement and regulations such as GEAR. The proposed new holding structures (LAB, specialty LFGs, and GEAR) were outlined, and discussed by the Head of Education with clinical and educational colleagues within KSS as part of the consultation process. This approach was well received, and it was agreed that these initiatives should be taken forward and implemented. In line with our process-consultancy approach, this led to a series of consultative workshops during the implementation period.

The purpose of the LAB was to oversee the academic and educational work of all the LFGs within its remit. Thus, there could be between eight and ten LFGs reporting to any given LAB in an LEP. The LAB was chaired by the local DME, and each LFG chair sat on the board, along with the local MEM, whose crucial pivotal role thus increasingly became closer to that of an Academic Registrar in a university. There was also funding to support a new role, that of Faculty Administrators; these Administrators worked with each LFG, and reported to the MEM. GEAR was mapped to national regulatory standards and, together with the LAB and LFG infrastructure, comprised LEP quality control for PGME in KSS. This innovative practice was recognised by the regulatory body, PMETB (now GMC), which commented in a visit to KSS in May (2009, 2) that:

> The Deanery has clearly mapped its expectations of local education providers (LEPs) against the PMETB domains through its Graduate Education and Assessment Regulations (GEAR) structure. This structure of local academic boards (LABs) and local faculty groups (LFGs) is ideally placed to monitor all aspects of patient safety both at trust level, and in the reporting arrangements to the Deanery.

## *Consultant Education Advisers for LFGs*

The third initiative was to support the embedding of all specialty LFGs. To this end we recruited, on a consultancy basis, seven senior education professionals, who had worked within mainstream higher education, and were very familiar with quality-assurance processes within such settings. Members of this group were called the Consultant Education Advisers [CEAs]. Each had responsibility for working in partnership with the LAB and LFGs in two LEPs. CEAs worked with LFG chairs, MEMs and Faculty Administrators to support and develop LFG practice locally. They negotiated entry into the LEP carefully, by discussing their role with LFG chairs and MEMs. Their main task was to attend each LFG in their LEP, to work with the LFG Chair and MEM to establish the common frameworks required by GEAR, and to support the LFG by identifying local good practice and issues for LFG development.

Prior to starting work in the field, we had identified a core of common generic LFG outcomes, which provided a benchmark for local discussions with the LFGs. These comprised, for example, ascertaining to what extent the LFG processes met the requirements of GEAR; whether postgraduate doctor progress was monitored by the LFG; and whether there were postgraduate doctor representatives on the LFG, who gave feedback on the quality of their PGME on behalf of their cohort. The CEAs were well aware of the delicacy of their position, and we discussed as a team how best to negotiate their entry into the field. Following Wenger (1998), we considered the delicacy of introducing into one practice, PGME, elements from the practice of another culture, HEI. We also discussed the need for the CEAs to be able to adopt a 'brokering' position, where their legitimacy to enter this new field of PGME was both recognised and mandated. The CEAs needed to be able to take up their role with authority, and also, as educationists, needed to signal their willingness to learn from clinicians and other professionals with whom they were working.

## LFG Action Plans and Emerging Practice

The involvement of the CEAs served not only to support the emerging LFGs, but also bore witness to the increasingly effective uptake of these initiatives. After attending LFG meetings, each CEA wrote an LFG Developmental Action Plan, which was sent to the LFG Chair, DME, and MEM for agreement and dissemination, before being shared within KSS with the Head of School appropriate to that specialty. The Plan was subsequently discussed with other CEAs on their regular development days. The Developmental Action Plans for each LFG identified good practice, action points, and points for development. Over a one-year period some 140 LFG Developmental Action Plans were written by the CEAs, and shared with the respective LFGs. There were numerous examples of emerging good practice. One CEA said that the style and manner in which the LFGs had been conducted had been important. Those conducted in an open and supportive environment were the most productive. She wrote:

> In nearly all cases, LFGs involve their trainees in such a way as to make them part of the specialty team. Their views are listened to, and I have personally witnessed numerous cases whereby trainee suggestions resolve rota difficulties and other operational and training issues.

Another CEA discussing what worked well in LFGs identified:

> meetings that are effectively chaired, and involve trainee representatives . . . these are very effective as they encourage pro-activeness and contributions to problem-solving. Time is used effectively, and there is encouragement to wrestle with seemingly intractable problems.

A further CEA noted:

> It was only because all Educational Supervisors were present at the LFG, that the discussion around one of the trainees resulted in their being formally identified as a Trainee in Difficulty. This is because the trainee had been cause for some minor concerns with one Educational Supervisor, and only because

he expressed this did two other Educational Supervisors confirm that they had, in fact, similar concerns. It then appeared that there were some specific family issues which may have impacted on this trainee. This then resulted in a lengthy discussion and agreement that the trainee would be seen the next day, the *Trainee in Difficulty Guidelines* would be followed, and further support be put in place.

One CEA commented on the LFG's 'active discussion' and 'willingness to develop the curriculum and introduce new opportunities for further training'. The CEA continued:

> A trainee at one Trust came very well prepared to the LFG with a summary of a trainee feedback pro forma, which was circulated to the LFG. This document gave a clear summary of trainees' views under the headings: Induction; teaching both formal and informal; service v training commitments; on calls and assessment processes; and educational and IT resources. This was a balanced account, and was well received by the meeting.

Another CEA noted the significant contribution that the MEMs and the Faculty Administrator made to the LFG, and commented on:

> the very active involvement of MEMs and Faculty Administrators . . . the MEMs contributed very effectively, especially where practice at the LFG was initially less sound. They support LFG Chairs well through subtle prompts about procedures.

A senior MEM, reflecting on the change process of recent years and the introduction of LFGs, LABs, and GEAR, commented that:

> the whole process has been brilliant. It puts a structure round what we do: for example, the progress of doctors in their training year. We didn't always hear about how they were doing, now it's more transparent . . . looking at trainee performance, I think it's excellent.

# Ways Forward: an Infrastructure for KSS

I have described how, working in partnership with those most committed to PGME within LEPs, we considered ways to build on existing practice in order to accommodate the new and evolving curricula and requirements. We worked and consulted with a group of key stakeholders as we set about establishing an infrastructure for local educational governance structures in each LEP or LFGs for each specialty, reporting to LABs. This consultative approach was also congruent with the professional conversation that we see as being at the heart of the Education Department's practice. We wanted to celebrate the importance of professional conversations as a dialogue with colleagues, attentive to complex, messy situations in practice. In these conversations, we were looking for local solutions to complex issues, thus offering the LEP opportunities for devolved educational autonomy.

Arising out of a process consultancy and partnership model, local creativity and problem-solving were supported, as were professional judgement and deliberation. Thus, the operational strategy has been one of enabling PGME 'not to be lost in translation, but held in transition', through conversations in practice within a series of organisational holding frames (LABs, LFGs, and GEAR), nested within a loosely coupled organisational structure. In this way, our process-consultancy approach sought to affirm the professional judgement of consultants as teachers, by offering further opportunities for the development of LEP communities of practice. We endeavoured to provide holding structures that would contain the change process, as Krantz (2001) has described. We were appreciative of the amount of time required for the change process, and the need for genuine, on-going investment in organisational roles, responsibilities, and structures.

The success of the change process is currently evident in the way in which the LFGs and LABs are evolving. We see considerable evidence of LEPs now taking firm ownership of these holding structures. In line with the Education Department's wish to support local creativity, we see LABs being further shaped by local stakeholders, DMEs, MEMs, LFG Chairs, and Faculty Administrators. LABs are becoming more congruent with individual LEP educational vision, educational governance, and authority, as well as continuing to meet the requirements of regulatory bodies. We also see professional deliberation, judgement, and accountability in support of postgraduate doctors and their PGME as a crucial bedrock for patient safety.

# References

Academy of Medical Royal Colleges Foundation Programme Committee. 2010. *UK Foundation Programme Curriculum 2010*. UK Foundation Programme Office: Cardiff.

Benjamin, J. 2004. Beyond the Doer and the Done to: An Inter-subjective View of Thirdness. *Psycho-Analytic Quarterly* 73 (1): 5-42.

Cooper, A. and T. Dartington. 2004. The Vanishing Organisation: Organisational Containment in a Networked World. In *Working below the surface: The Emotional Life of Contemporary Organisations*, eds. C. Huffington, D. Armstrong, W. Halton, L. Hoyle and J. Pooley, 127-150. Tavistock Clinic Series. London: Karnac.

Eraut, M. 2008. *Evaluation of the Introduction of the Intercollegiate Surgical Curriculum Project*. London: Royal College of Surgeons.

Grant, J. 2009. *Moral Panic, Political Imperative and What the Profession Knows About Developing its New Generations*. Plenary Address. The Association for Medical Education Europe. 1 September 2009.

Hirschhorn, L. 1997. *Reworking Authority: Leading and Following in the Post-Modern Organisation*. Cambridge: MIT.

Krantz, J. 2001. Dilemmas of Organisational Change. *In The Systems Psycho-dynamics of Organisations*, eds. Gould, L., L. Stapley, M. Stein, 133-156. London: Karnac.

KSS Education Department. 2010. *Graduate Education and Assessment Regulations*. 3rd edition. London: KSS Deanery.

MacIntyre, A. 1981. *After Virtue: A Study in Moral Theory.* London: Duckworth.

Modernising Medical Careers. 2009. *Maintaining Quality of Training in a Reduced Training Opportunity Environment*. Paper 21-7. London: MMC.

Moss, F. 1995. Rethinking Consultants: Alternative Models of Organisation are Needed. *BMJ*. 310: 925. 8 April 1995.

PMETB 2009. *Report to KSS Deanery 2009*. PMETB: London.

Schein, E. H. 1988. *Process Consultation, Volume 1*. Wokingham: Addison Wesley.

Schein, E.H. 1990. A General Philosophy of Helping: Process Consultation. *Sloan Management Review*. 31. (3): 57-64.

Wenger, E. 1998. *Communities of Practice: Learning, Meaning and Identity*. Cambridge: CUP.

# Part Two:

## Journeys in Postgraduate Medical Education

# The KSS Qualified Educational Supervisor Programme

## Principles and Values

> I certainly find my mind opened to more varied ways of teaching that once
> tried have been more effective than the didactic instructive methods that
> I find tempting when I feel pushed for time or there's a lot to cover (QESP
> evaluation from a Gastroenterology surgeon).

The Qualified Educational Supervisor Programme [QESP] is an innovative and unique programme developed by the Education Department at Kent, Surrey and Sussex Postgraduate Medical Deanery [KSS] over a period of seventeen years. QESP was an early expression of the Education Department's 'principled approach to practice', described in Chapter 2, and it remains a fundamental part of our work. I lead QESP, and most of our Assistant Deans in Education [ADEs] spend some of their time teaching it. However, QESP is taught predominantly by a team of nineteen part-time Consultant Education Advisers [CEAs], who are drawn from mainstream higher education.

The aim of QESP is to help clinicians to reflect on, and to develop, their educational practices. QESP itself is practice-based since, as Elliott (2001, 123) says, 'what constitutes an appropriate realisation of human value must be judged in situ rather than standardised and routinised'. The majority of QESP takes place in the real-life contexts of clinical teaching and educational supervision, and so must take into account constraints such as the reduction in teaching time for postgraduate medical education [PGME], created by the European Working Time Regulations [EWTR].

QESP's focus on individual development, and its explicitly stated principles and values, mean that it has more in common with mainstream teacher education than with the 'Train the Trainers' programmes that typify medical education. However, in many ways, QESP runs counter to much contemporary mainstream education, since we do not impose pre-specified objectives, we do not measure performance against checklists, and there is no competency base. QESP is work-based but not vocational. Using the distinction made in Chapter 2, QESP offers education, not training; it seeks to develop the whole person, rather than trying to ensure 'that the same reaction is always given to a similar event' (de Cossart and Fish 2005, 46). Within the programme, we aim to support clinicians in the development of a particular set of 'characteristics' that have been developed collaboratively by CEAs and ADEs (Figure 1). These characteristics, which underpin our work, reflect our experience of working with doctors in real-life clinical settings, such as theatres, clinics, and on ward-rounds. They provide descriptive statements of the development we would expect to see in successful QESP participants. At the same time, they avoid a 'one size fits all' approach by seeking to respect the varied and creative ways in which doctors combine PGME with the 'service' demands of the National Health Service [NHS]. KSS doctors find that this combination of a values-based approach with one-to-one teaching in their real-life clinical workplace, is very helpful to them.

QESP is popular with potential teachers as well as with learners; on one round of recruitment, over a hundred people applied to become CEAs. Applicants express particular interest in QESP's clear, ethical value-base; its refusal of reductive checklists; its use of a professional conversation rather than feedback; and its real-life clinical contexts. The programme also represents value for money. Although we employ highly experienced CEAs, with an immense range and depth of experience in education, and especially in teacher education, most of QESP takes place at the participant's place of work. This minimises disruption to clinical service, avoids locum costs, and removes travel costs for participants, thereby providing financial efficiency as well as educational effectiveness.

The programme is organised in two parts, QESP Part 1 (the Certificate in Teaching), and QESP Part 2 (the Certificate in Educational Supervision). First of all, I shall explain how the programme works in practice. Then, I shall look in more detail at the professional conversations that form the main part of QESP, and consider whether these conversations develop a third space between those participating in them.

(ↀ)

# Characteristics of an Educational Supervisor

'Sound teaching makes safe doctors'. These statements constitute a summary of the characteristics we aim to develop on the KSS Qualified Educational Supervisor Programme (Parts 1 and 2).

## Qualified Educational Supervisor Programme: Part 1

- A developing awareness of their own educational principles and values
- Willingness to reflect on and adapt their own educational practice and to engage in professional conversation
- Interest in some of the complexities of their role as educators in clinical settings
- Interest in some of the complexities of learning and assessment
- Ability to recognise and adapt to learners' individual learning needs and levels of competence and confidence
- Awareness of the educational value of role modelling, and of themselves as role models
- Ability to contribute to the development of a learning environment where individual differences are respected and valued
- Engagement with curriculum change and assessment processes
- Recognising the importance of collaborative and team work in reflective educational practice

As part of this process, they are likely also to have thought about and developed further the following areas:

- A developing awareness of a range of teaching methodologies and underpinning principles
- Ability to articulate their educational position
- Moving from a focus on teaching towards a focus on learning
- Establishing a supportive learning environment
- Finding ways to encourage learners to notice more in clinical settings
- Recognising the value of tolerating uncertainty
- Finding ways to make expectations and learning opportunities explicit
- Being open to learner participation, shifting the balance of power between teacher and learner
- Making explicit their own thinking and uncertainties

Figure 1: Characteristics of an Educational Supervisor

---

## Qualified Educational Supervisor Programme: Part 2

- Ability to foster learners' autonomy
- Ability to convey clear and principled expectations
- Ability to collaborate with colleagues in order to monitor and support learners' progression
- Understanding of the range of learning, assessment and support opportunities available in clinical settings
- Engagement with the changing structures and processes of medical and academic curricula, assessment and careers
- Awareness of and engagement with local processes of educational governance
- Ability and willingness to use local processes in order to champion the specific needs of learners and their supervisors, with attention to patient safety.

---

Figure 1: Characteristics of an Educational Supervisor.

## The Programme in Practice

### QESP Part 1: the Certificate in Teaching

Part 1 of QESP begins with a workshop entitled *Principles and Values in Education*. The purpose of the workshop is to introduce participants to the processes for the Certificate in Teaching, and to help them to begin to explore and reflect on educational practices. The intention is also that participants begin to talk together about some of their underlying assumptions and values. Rather than merely affirming these existing assumptions, we hope that the workshop discussions will, if anything, have an unsettling effect, and will support participants in becoming more curious about teaching and learning, and in beginning to see education as a complex activity, worthy of considerable exploration.

The workshop does not set out to give simple answers about complex educational processes. Its purpose is not to provide tips about teaching, or to tell consultants how to teach. Its underlying principle is that participants need to do their own learning, by using and applying new ideas, whatever teaching methods they choose. Barnes calls this 'the learner "working on understanding"' in order to 'reorganise his or her existing pictures of the world' (Barnes 1992, 124). Thus, QESP facilitates thinking and reflection, in whatever way seems most helpful to each participant. This educational support can be characterised as 'walking alongside' the participant, or as offering 'scaffolding' to support the candidate's development of their own educational thinking (Bruner 1966; Mercer 2000).

During the workshop we ask participants to engage in a range of activities, in order to help them to reflect on their experience, and to challenge their practice, and their assumptions. These activities include asking them to choose a quotation about education from a selection provided, and then to talk about their reasons for choosing it. Quotations which are popular with participants include: 'thought only starts with doubt', 'getting it wrong is part of getting it right', and 'education is the lighting of a fire, not the filling of a pail'. These quotations prompt rich, varied, and engaged discussions by participants about practical, and philosophical, aspects of teaching and learning in their particular clinical contexts.

In the workshop we also discuss participants' concerns, such as assessing postgraduate doctors, and teaching in their clinical workplaces. Participants are encouraged to consider what particular aspects of their teaching they would like to explore with their CEA during the one-to-one visits, in order to develop their practice. Starting points for these future explorations are often questions prompted by participation in the workshop.

QESP workshop participants are drawn from a range of Local Education Providers [LEPs], and so one group usually includes a range of specialties, such as Paediatrics, Surgery, Elderly Medicine, Obstetrics and Gynaecology, Palliative Care, and Psychiatry. Each specialty and sub-specialty sees itself as having distinct educational issues that are quite separate from the educational issues of other specialties. However, having worked with clinicians from all specialties, we note a range of concerns and issues that they hold in common. For instance, although community-based psychiatrists may see their concerns as being very different from those of surgeons, both groups are likely to be: balancing 'service delivery' with educational activity; supporting less experienced colleagues in providing good patient care; teaching history taking; teaching about patient consent; and dealing with organisational management issues.

Participants often appear uncomfortable and anxious when they arrive at the workshop, but usually leave feeling enthusiastic about the programme. This change in perception is epitomised by one cardiologist, who wrote on the evaluation form, 'I have to say that, despite initially feeling very apprehensive and anxious about today's encounter, the final experience in many ways was extremely encouraging and uplifting'.

After the initial workshop, each participant is allocated a CEA, who negotiates the first of a minimum of three visits. We encourage participants to arrange to be visited and observed when they are engaged in their regular educational activities, and to see their CEA as a resource to help with teaching in real-life *clinical* settings, rather than formal lectures, although the latter are not precluded. During visits, the CEA will usually make observations, not judgements, and will write notes in a narrative style to a timeline, attempting to capture much of what has been said during the observed session. A copy of the written notes is given to the participant. Immediately after each observed session, the CEA and the participant have an hour's one-to-one professional conversation in a private location chosen by the participant.

As soon as possible after this conversation, participants are asked to write brief reflective notes, which can be seen as a continuation of the conversation, and which may help the CEA to further understand what the visit has meant to the participant. This can be built on and developed in subsequent visits. The following extract from a surgeon's reflections on his teaching shows something of the quality of his learning through this process:

> I tried questions like 'what might you do?', 'what if?', 'what do you think of?', and 'would it be a good idea' rather than sharp, shooting, spotlight questions that seem a bit like weapons to a stressed, junior audience. It seemed more effective in eliciting a thoughtful response and, at the time, I thought, there were fewer pauses in our conversation. More two-way, definitely. Certainly, we covered the same amount of material but seemed to finish with time to spare.

At least two further visits are made, and more may be made by agreement, until both the participant and their CEA are content that the participant's educational practice is satisfactory.

## QESP Part 2: the Certificate in Educational Supervision

Part 2 of QESP sets out to help participants clarify the differences between the roles of a clinical and an educational supervisor, and to reflect this distinction in their practice. It focuses on the supervision of postgraduate doctors' educational progress, including assessment, careers support, and supporting postgraduate doctors with additional learning needs. Part 2 extends the application of the principles and practice learned in Part 1 to the specific context of educational supervision. Typically, Part 2 is completed over a period of three to four months.

Part 2 also starts with a workshop, where participants are encouraged to reflect on and share ideas arising from their experience of Part 1. Typical examples of their comments are:

> The course was reassuring – usually no-one gets to see you teaching in a clinic.

> It was fascinating – I learned to empathise with the trainee.

> I learned not to do all the work for the trainees in teaching, talking, or telling. I was helped to ask myself 'do I talk too much?'

> I realised that teaching and learning is not necessarily formally structured – but that I can formalise what learning has occurred. I recognised that learning by doing is teaching – and therefore also valuable for the trainee.

> I recognised that we learn by teaching – so it's valuable for trainees to be put into a teaching or telling position

Participants consider a range of issues relevant to educational supervision, such as: clarifying and mapping the role of an Educational Supervisor, in terms of principles, values, and practices; supporting postgraduate doctors' use of portfolios; developing reflective talk and writing; overseeing workplace-based assessment; and giving effective and constructive feedback. They are given information and support in relation to advising on medical careers, and helping postgraduate doctors with additional learning needs. A course booklet offers further readings on supervision and related educational issues. Viewing and discussion of a locally filmed DVD showing a supervision session offers participants the chance to raise uncertainties about the process, to share their ideas and experiences, and to learn through hearing the ideas of others. QESP Part 2 workshops are usually composed of consultants at different stages in their own learning about the role of supervisor, and so they provide a valuable opportunity for peers to share practice. To encourage reflection on practice, a model of working one-to-one with postgraduate doctors is presented in the form of a role-played, professional conversation.

The workshop is followed by a minimum of two observations of the participant working as an Educational Supervisor. As in Part 1 of QESP, each observation is followed by an hour's professional conversation, informed by the CEA's observation notes. Reflective comments are exchanged between participant and adviser by email between each visit, again with the aim of extending the professional conversation, and the process of reflection, between visits.

There is also the possibility for participants to undertake voluntary, reciprocated peer observations. Those who have taken the time to take part in these observations have found them particularly helpful.

## Evaluation and Development

Our practice is to evaluate each workshop, and to review each part of QESP on an ongoing basis, asking participants for qualitative feedback. This informs our practice and our planning for the future. The following, very brief, selection of comments represents the thoughtful appreciation we often receive, and goes some way towards illustrating the aspects of the course most frequently mentioned by participants:

> [My CEA] was very supportive and gave some constructive criticism, with evidence-base to allow me to further look at my practice. I would strongly advise my colleagues with an interest in improving their teaching and to know what they are doing is based in fact, to attend this course. A very positive experience (consultant radiologist).
>
> I felt more reassured than challenged (not a bad feeling to be left with!) (consultant physician).
>
> I felt more confident about my teaching methods and gained useful insight into my teaching and how to improve it (consultant oncologist).
>
> They [my learners] learn more if stretched but not too stressed. I am doing some things right! (consultant physician).

It is now a General Medical Council [GMC] requirement for Educational Supervisors to be accredited (GMC 2010, 30). Some Postgraduate Medical Deaneries [Deaneries] are meeting this national requirement by using e-learning, and classroom-based courses. Other Deaneries have expressed interest in the practice-based nature of the work of QESP, and are interested in moving from a classroom-based competency model, towards supporting reflection through professional conversation. Mapped against the Academy of Medical Educators' *Professional Standards* (AoME 2009), QESP meets, and in some areas exceeds, the standards for level 1, thus demonstrating that it goes well beyond the national mandatory minimum required by the GMC.

## Professional Conversations

> In our last conversation you told me not to mouth the answers to my
> questions to the students! (consultant neurologist).

I should now like to explore the value of 'professional conversations' as spaces for reflection on teaching and learning, that is, as dialogues, creating opportunities for educational development. In this exploration I shall draw on examples of my professional conversations with hospital consultants on QESP. When I have these conversations, I set out to create a 'third space' between the clinical world of the hospital consultant, and my educational world, where we can discuss our shared experience of the observation, and where 'alternative and competing discourses and positionings transform conflict and difference into rich zones of collaboration and learning' (Gutierrez et al 2003, 171).

I am particularly interested in the negotiation of a curriculum through conversations between CEA and QESP participant. This reflects my interest in the ways in which teachers may negotiate and develop understandings, by taking into account the individual needs of learners. The professional conversation is an opportunity for teacher and learner – CEA and clinician, in this case – to share and develop understandings of what is educationally possible and desirable within a specific context. The view I shall present is that professional conversations that are jointly negotiated, or co-constructed, may be more effective than a traditional feedback model, in which the teacher's agenda is predominant, and the learner tends to be less actively involved.

My interest in conversations and learning dialogues stems from my experience as a teacher in state schools in the UK, and from my work with teachers in the National Oracy Project. Here I became convinced of the value of learner talk within group work. These professional experiences created a link with my own personal experience of preferring (and possibly *needing*) to make sense of things myself, by discussing, by arguing, by explaining, by exploring, and by trying out ideas, through talking with others. I was, I think, quite young, when I realised that most of us do not learn much by being told, or by being lectured at.

These approaches are in contrast to the way most classrooms (and other learning settings, meetings, and management groups) are run. Generally, it is the teacher (or the chair of the meeting, or the manager) who does most of the talking, and it is the others who, therefore, do most of the listening. Pradl (1988, 33) uses irony when he says, 'As teachers we naturally have much advice to give, much information to dispense. If only our students would listen to us, the educational puzzle would be solved once and for all'. He goes on to argue: 'To give someone something, even knowledge, means we will have to come to terms with the other person's outlook on our very act of giving'. Many teachers (or chairs of meetings, or managers) would espouse some of the theoretical principles briefly outlined in this chapter, and yet would probably find it hard to resist trying to do too much 'giving' through talking.

Most courses offered within PGME are 'run', 'presented', or 'delivered' – all terms that imply a transmission model of teaching, and a passive role for the learner. Many courses are taught in classrooms, rather than being based in the real-life messiness and busyness of clinical settings. PGME also places a strong emphasis on e-learning, which tends towards an individual or solitary model of learning, where it is assumed that 'one size fits all'.

By contrast, the emphasis in QESP on workplace-based observation means that we are able to see the specific difficulties that participants are dealing with, and that we can discuss these within the professional conversation. The challenge is then to use the shared context of an observed session, in order to support each participant in learning to develop their ability to reflect on their own educational practices. The QESP course document states that successful candidates will have shown and developed further their 'willingness to reflect on and adapt their own educational practice and to engage in professional conversation' (Figure 1).

I see professional conversations as a place where two people, the clinician and the CEA, can work together to negotiate a curriculum, to work on understandings, and to make meanings. In a professional conversation we aim to be open to what arises, since the outcome is unknown, and cannot be planned for, or predicted. Volosinov (1986, 102) says that, 'meaning is like an electric spark that occurs only when two different terminals are hooked together'. There is something of that 'spark' of meaning between different people in the most effective QESP conversations. The conversations do not usually take a clear linear direction; instead, they follow a path that loops and meanders between the participants, a path negotiated and traversed by both of them:

> We say that we 'conduct' a conversation, but the more genuine a conversation is, the less its conduct lies within the will of either partner. Thus a genuine conversation is never the one that we wanted to conduct. Rather, it is more generally correct to say that we fall into conversation, or even that we become involved in it. The way one word follows another, with conversation taking its own twists and reaching its own conclusion, may well be conducted in some way, but the partners conversing are far less the leaders of it than the led (Gadamer 1998, 383).

Thus it is in my professional conversations; I aim to be *involved* in them, rather than *conduct* them, or *lead* them. Part of my specific purpose is to avoid being 'teacherly' and didactic, and to attempt to bring my educational experience and understandings to meet the concerns and interests of the consultant. However, this is more difficult than it sounds! It means that the agenda of the conversation, and thus the curriculum of QESP, is negotiated within the conversations themselves. I set out with a clear focus on the general principles and values outlined in Chapter 2, and the specific features described in Figure 1, but the challenge is to ensure that those concerns support, rather than prevent, my ability to listen and to engage with my conversational partner.

My conversations and my development of QESP have been influenced by social constructivism, the idea that learning is essentially a social process of negotiated meanings. An important implication of this theory is that a transmission model of learning does not work, because learners need to engage in the learning process to construct their own understandings. As Douglas Barnes writes:

> Whatever teaching methods a teacher chooses – question and answer, guided discovery, demonstration, or another – it will always be the pupil who has to do the learning (Barnes 1992,124).

Helpfully, Barnes (1992, 125) offers us the phrase 'working on understanding', as a way of thinking about the actual *process*, rather than the *product*, of learning. Process is particularly important in QESP professional conversations, because participants come from very different professions and discourse communities. This may mean that we occupy different 'frames', (Goffman 1974) within the conversations. The consultants may expect assessment, feedback, and tips on teaching, while the CEAs tend to look for development, openness, and reflection. This is because, as Swann et al say, '"Frame" refers to our knowledge, based on previous experience, about the typical organisation of an event or activity' (Swann et al 2004,117). In my conversations I attempt to bridge discourses, to find and use common ground, and to create 'third spaces', in order to negotiate and develop shared understandings. As the conversations occur within workplace settings, and within 'the highly politicised contexts of PGME' (Chapter 2), they require the careful development and maintenance of trust between the two participants.

Within social constructivism, a 'discourse community' describes institutions that are brought into being through particular kinds of conversations and interactions. This indicates that language is constitutive, and that specific interactions are 'where meanings are created and changed' (Taylor 2001, 6). In these conversations, each individual needs to maintain and negotiate their personal and professional identities. The concepts of 'face' and 'face-work' (Goffman 1959) are relevant here in terms of how people manage their own and the other person's public self-image within interactions. These considerations point to the potential complications in professional conversations, which occur between two people from different discourse communities, and with complex power differentials. Both participants may be keen to preserve, or to challenge, their own and others' professional identities, and thereby to prove their own professional credibility.

∞

# Third Space

I conceive of the 'third space' as a place where people can feel safe to challenge, to think, to risk, and to begin to transform. This may involve people taking on new ways of being, talking, and understanding. Drawing on post-colonial theory (Bhabha 1994), another way to think of this is as a form of hybridity between different cultures: a space that spans the clinical and educational worlds which QESP participants and CEAs separately occupy. In QESP, the creation of a third space is dependent on both participants acting in a reciprocal manner, so that neither person takes on just one role as teacher or learner. Like everyday conversations, the aim is for the relationships within QESP professional conversations to be 'reversible and reflexive' (Burbules 1993, 82). Both CEAs and QESP participants need to be willing to listen and to learn, to be tentative and exploratory, and to be inquiring and wide-ranging.

Participants appear to approach the programme with different pedagogical expectations to those held by CEAs. Many participants write about their nervousness at having their teaching observed and discussed. Often, they mention this initial fear and anxiety in their reflections between visits, and in their final evaluations of the course. Some doctors write that they expect the course to be about picking up 'tips' on teaching. As Jason, a consultant cardiologist said, 'I initially entered the course thinking that my main objective was to learn the "rules" required to become an effective teacher'. Consultants often call us their assessors when introducing us to their teams, despite our referring to ourselves as their CEAs. These assumptions indicate the cultural differences that must be bridged and, indeed, in Chapter 2, Zoë Playdon describes educationists as 'guests in the world of medicine'. Many participants have had no previous opportunities to reflect formally on their teaching. Thus, the initial purposes of a professional conversation may be to reassure, to give voice, to make links, and ultimately to develop shared understandings.

So what might a third space look and sound like in professional conversation? I try to enable its creation through a balance of support and challenge, and by encouraging participants to explore their practice in an open and tentative way. There is a sense in which the whole aim of the professional conversation is to provide a third space in a macro sense, whilst the moment-by-moment exchanges within the conversation provide (or where less effective, can remove) a third space in a micro sense. This suggests a complex interplay, in which participants shift between understandings, whilst protecting and maintaining a sense of their identity within the conversation.

# Case Study: Looking for the Third Space in Practice

I recorded, transcribed, and analysed several sequences of professional conversations, including a set of three with 'Jason', a consultant cardiologist. I am going to refer to key moments from the conversations, where it would appear that there is evidence of a third space developing between us, and I will look at some of the factors that have helped bring these into being. In my transcriptions I keep punctuation to a minimum and include hesitations and pauses, as I am interested in participants' thinking, and hesitations, and other features of talk may provide evidence of this. All those involved, other than myself, have been anonymised.

My first example is the opening of the conversation with Jason. After brief comments regarding my recording equipment, I ask, 'Erm, ok, so how would you like to do this? Would you like to start off by saying how you thought that went? Or would you like me to start off erm with some of my kind of observations and questions?' My aim in asking this question is to share the agenda of the conversation, aiming to find out more about the candidate's understandings, and the issues he would like to explore, and to support him in thinking and reflecting. Although I am leading the opening of the conversation, I sound tentative and offer the option of starting with 'my kind of observations and questions'. This is an example of my attempting to mitigate the potential challenge of the question by suggesting that there are alternatives, and thus offering opportunities for face-saving.

Jason responds by rephrasing my question, which may be for clarification, or might be a delaying tactic. He says, 'Erm how did it go? I, I can start for a little bit', thus signalling a mixture of willingness and uncertainty. He continues, 'I mean in a way that is very much a typical round and the ECG of the day that that's how it's been most of the time'. He is signalling that this observed practice is 'in a way', 'very much', or 'most of the time' normal practice, and yet these hedges may serve to either protect him from appearing to boast, or may be attempting to hide the fact that this is not in fact 'typical' practice.

I ask him a challenging question: 'And you'd normally spend as long as that on the ECG of the day?' What I had observed after the ward-round was an unusually long period of time being given to an explicit teaching session. My question aims to find out whether this is something that usually happens, or whether it has been set up because of my presence. Jason responds at length. He appears to show that he has heard the implied challenge to his 'face' because he says in reply, regarding the ECG teaching session, 'You know I'm not saying we staged that . . . ', which suggests an element of justification and explanation on his part.

In the exchanges at the opening of this first conversation, Jason articulates some of his interests and concerns about his teaching. For example, he says, 'I quite like knowing what they're going to talk about because it allows me then to just do a bit of reading around it', indicating that he likes to be in the position of expert. He also says, 'Sometimes I feel that I have too much and I can't quite restrain myself in delivering it and I think that probably one of my big problems is, is not being able to restrain once they let the draw you know the draw gates up you know I'm sort of, bluh it all comes out', suggesting that he thinks he has a tendency to talk too much.

These comments form a foundation for the rest of the conversation and, indeed, for future conversations. Moreover, they begin to establish a feeling of trust, where concerns can be raised and heard. I respond to Jason's comment about talking too much by asking: 'And why do you think that's a problem potentially?' and he replies: 'Well because I probably think that it doesn't allow a erm structure to the development of an argument about something I mean maybe not I don't know erm and I might go a bit too fast and they might not be able to keep up'. This tells me that he understands something of the need for teachers to encourage, rather than prevent, learners' active engagement, which is the foundation of an understanding of social constructivist theory. We return to this point on other occasions, for example during our second conversation, where Jason acknowledges the need for learners to develop understanding through talking things through: 'You might do it internally but it doesn't seem to solidify it so much unless you vocalise it'.

A later conversation with Jason shows something of the continuing development of his ability to articulate his educational thinking. Following the observation of an outpatient clinic, he again appears to feel able to raise his concerns, saying early on: 'Why do I always feel . . . that I fall short you know of delivering a good experience to the people that I teach?' In asking this question he is returning to a comment he had made in the initial workshop, where he had expressed the opinion that some people shouldn't teach (and therefore shouldn't have postgraduate doctors) because they're not good at it. Jason was referring to himself. My replies, both in the workshop and in this professional conversation, indicated my belief that doubting one's ability as a teacher may indicate a willingness to reflect on the learner's needs, and also to develop as a teacher.

In this third conversation, Jason remembers and applies topics from previous conversations, in a way that demonstrates his reflexivity. He says, in response to my question towards the end, 'I feel satisfied that we've covered things in a way', and asks 'do you think there's anything more?', but then says that he feels 'that you've provoked enough thought in me'. When I suggest 'and I think you've done most of that for yourself' he replies 'yeah no no you've facilitated that that's what it's all about isn't it?'. This suggests that he has noticed aspects of the way that we have worked together, and the interpersonal and ideational model that I have provided. Is Jason suggesting that this 'facilitation' is a form of third space? The tentative, exploratory way in which we have both been able to approach Jason's concerns felt, at times, like the development of a third space, and a 'zone of collaboration and learning' (Gutierrez et al, 2003).

## An Elusive Concept

I find the concept of the creation of third spaces in professional conversations tantalising. Rather like looking for learning, once one looks for it actually occurring in real time, in the process of coming into being, it is elusive. For the conversations to be effective, both participants need to enter and inquire into the frame of the other, while thinking aloud, reflecting, using tentative, exploratory talk, and listening to the other. Where this does not happen, a third space is either not developed, or is not maintained, and so disappears.

For example, the first conversation with Nita, a consultant paediatrician, took place after a morning handover meeting and a long ward-round, during which an incident occurred where a registrar had hurt and upset a child. Initially Nita said very little, resisting my invitation for her to take a lead, and letting me do all the talking, but after a few minutes she said,

'Particularly with that registrar that we had on the ward-round today certain expectations I had of him that erm you know I felt that he should have fulfilled'. This is tentative, relative to much of Nita's speech, and possibly indicates her risking raising a topic that she would like to explore. She has responded to my question about differentiating teaching, and has entered my educational frame, by raising an issue that had come up on the ward-round, in a half-tentative ('erm you know'), and half-definite way ('certain expectations I had of him' and 'he should have fulfilled'). I think it may have felt to Nita that she had risked her professional 'face' by raising this issue, as she is not articulating a clear position here. Unfortunately, I do not use this opportunity to enter her frame of clinical concern, regarding what can be expected of a registrar, and this opportunity to discuss the issue raised by her is not then revisited until much later in the conversation. When analysing the dialogue, I was left wondering why I did not appear to hear her concern and why I did not enter her frame earlier, possibly using a tentative, exploratory tone myself. I also wondered what the effects on this and subsequent conversations with her might have been, if I had done so. As it was, it took until towards the end of the third conversation for it to feel as though there was trust between us, and an elusive and fragile third space was finally established.

Crucially, the concept of a third space, and the practice of professional conversations, like all teaching and learning encounters, require reciprocity. As Burbules (1993, 21) says:

> the dialogical encounter engages the participants in a process at once symbiotic and synergistic; beyond a particular point, no one may be consciously guiding or directing it, and the order and flow of the communicative exchange itself takes over. The participants are caught up; they are absorbed.

The curriculum of the professional conversations is focused in part by the characteristics listed in Figure 1. More importantly, the agenda and topics of the conversations are negotiated within the conversations themselves. For example, a regular topic of my professional conversations, such as those with Jason, is learner engagement in their learning. However, this topic is not *introduced* by me, but picked up from his comments about talking too much, and we appear to move together into the topic of learner engagement. In other words, the topics themselves are co-constructed in the to-and-fro of the conversation.

Thus, the co-construction of a curriculum, or agenda, within the professional conversation, means that the development needs of the QESP participant can be explored within this space. The conversations need to be co-constructed through attentive listening and face-work, where each person responds to the other, and both participants make joint reference to the shared context of the observation, in order for both to be 'caught up' and 'absorbed'.

Such a creation of a third space is necessary in settings where there is a meeting of people from different discourse communities, with potentially different expectations. It must, however, be remembered that third spaces need careful creation and maintenance, through extremely sensitive engagement in professional conversations.

# References

Academy of Medical Educators. 2009. *Professional Standards*. London: Academy of Medical Educators.

Barnes, D. 1992. The Role of Talk in Learning. In *Thinking Voices*, ed. K. Norman, 123-128. London: Hodder and Stoughton.

Bhabha, H. 1994. *The Location of Culture*. London: Routledge.

Bruner, J. 1966. *Towards a Theory of Instruction*. Harvard: Belknap Press.

Burbules, N. 1993. Dialogue in Teaching. *Theory and Practice*. New York: Teachers College Press.

de Cossart, L., and D. Fish, 2005. *Cultivating a Thinking Surgeon*. Shrewsbury, tfm Publishing.

Elliott, J. 2001. *Action Research for Educational Change*. Milton Keynes: Open University Press.

Gadamer, H. G. 1998. *Truth and Method*. New York: Continuum.

General Medical Council. 2010. *Quality Framework Operational Guide*: Supplementary Guidance. London: GMC.

Goffman, E. 1959. *The Presentation of Self in Everyday Life*. New York: Doubleday Anchor.

Goffman, E., 1974, *Frame Analysis*. Harmondsworth: Penguin.

Gutierrez, C., P. Baquedano-Lopez and C. Tejeda. 2003. Rethinking Diversity: Hybridity and Hybrid Language Practices in the Third Space. In *Language, Literacy and Education: A Reader,* eds. S. Goodman, T.Lillis, J. Maybin and N. Mercer, 286-303. Stoke on Trent: Trentham Books.

Mercer, N. 2000. *Words and Minds*. London: Routledge.

Pradl, G. 1988. Learning Listening. In *The Word for Teaching is Learning: Essays for James Britton*, eds. M. Lightfoot and N. Martin, 33-48. Oxford: Heinemann.

Swann, J., A. Deumert, T. Lillis and R. Mesthrie, 2004. *A Dictionary of Sociolinguistics*. Edinburgh: Edinburgh University Press.

Taylor, S. 2001. Locating and Conducting Discourse Analytic Research. In *Discourse as Data*, eds. M. Wetherell, S. Taylor, and S. Yates, 5-48. London: Sage.

Volosinov, V.1986. *Marxism and the Philosophy of Language*. Cambridge: Harvard University Press.

# Educational Supervision: a Narrative Approach

## Do Stories Have a Place in Educational Supervision?

I have worked as an Assistant Dean Education [ADE] at Kent, Surrey and Sussex Postgraduate Medical Deanery [KSS] for several years. Formerly I was a secondary English teacher in the state sector and then a university lecturer and teacher educator, working mainly with postgraduates preparing for a profession in teaching. My years at KSS have represented an extraordinarily rich opportunity for learning, and in this chapter I have recorded and started to reflect on some of what I have learned, specifically in my role as course leader for the KSS Qualified Educational Supervisor Programme [QESP] Part 2: the Certificate in Educational Supervision.

From my perspective, much of what is currently happening in postgraduate medical education [PGME] looks like a familiar story of educational upheaval and change. Along with this comes the perennial need for teachers to retain the best of what we already know and value, while making the best of whatever new comes our way. As a non-clinician, my understandings in this context will always be partial. I write from a liminal position, looking in through doors that have been opened by the generous clinicians I have encountered in this work, and with a foot in my own past and my own learning story.

Working with beginning teachers and their school mentors, I often found that what both needed was a chance to reflect on how best a professional at the start of their career may learn 'on the job' in a very busy working environment. For me, working out *how* to learn has been an essential part of learning, and I see the exchange of stories as an effective way to develop such thinking, affording proper attention to the complexity of the learning process and its often serendipitous nature in workplace settings. I suggest that a narrative approach to educational supervision in PGME invites Educational Supervisors to give postgraduate doctors a chance to tell the story of their learning – and in the telling, to own it more fully and perhaps to change it.

## Changing Language: Changing Stories

As a result of the changes required by the national report on *Modernising Medical Careers* (2005), and as discussed in detail in Chapter 3, new, highly structured and explicit National Curriculum Frameworks [NCFs] have been introduced for postgraduate doctors. In KSS, these NCFs are in the process of being mapped within our Local Education Providers [LEPs] to ensure that their requirements are met by the learning provided in the workplace. The introduction of NCFs and the accompanying process of creating a Local Curriculum in Practice [LCP] have heralded significant changes in educational processes and in the language of PGME. As Vygotsky (1962) demonstrated, thought and language are very closely interconnected, so that language performs a mediating function in intellectual development. Changes in language in this sense mediate our understandings. They become a determining factor in the ways in which we are able to think.

The current terms for 'learning' and 'learners' in PGME are 'training' and 'trainees', which now replace the even more old-fashioned 'apprenticeship' and 'junior doctors'. These terms are accompanied by other similar terminology, such as 'trainee portfolios' and assessment 'tools' which require the measurement of 'performance' against lists of 'competencies'. These replace a former language, one that reflected a different emphasis, namely an emphasis on clinical practice, which placed trust in the ability of clinicians to make their own, more holistic judgements on the progress of 'junior doctors' in their care, and to mediate these judgements within a small local community of practice, the medical 'firm'. Perhaps these changes in language also change doctors' perceptions of the kinds of stories it is possible to tell as part of the process of teaching and learning. In KSS, we refer to doctors undertaking postgraduate education as 'postgraduate doctors', rather than as 'juniors' or 'trainees'. 'Juniors' has potentially patronising connotations when applied to professionals at an advanced stage in their continuing education, and 'trainees' suggests a limiting and mechanistic view of education.

## The Value of Educational Supervision

> 'Have you ever talked to your own trainees about the way you learned?'
> 'No, I don't think so. This is the first time I've ever talked to anyone about it.'
> (from a conversation with a consultant anaesthetist on the KSS Certificate in Educational Supervision [QESP], 2008).

Many of the clinicians involved in teaching postgraduate doctors acknowledge the usefulness of more explicit curricula. NCFs have paid close attention to those areas of 'episteme' or propositional knowledge so necessary to postgraduate doctors. In theory, chance now plays a smaller part in the vital matter of ensuring that new doctors will have at their fingertips all the knowledge and skills necessary in order to practise in contemporary clinical contexts. However, as researchers and educationists Della Fish and Linda de Cossart have identified, there is within 'a profession accustomed to adapting fast to new enterprises

. . . an all-pervasive disquiet' (Fish and de Cossart 2007, 10). In my work at KSS, I have come into contact with this disquiet as well as strong sense, among many doctors who are committed to improving their own educational practice, that precious elements of teaching and learning in clinical settings are in danger of being lost. There is a sense that in 'the naming of parts', something of great value has been dismantled, and that the way to reassemble it has been lost. As Richard Sennett has commented, 'When an institution like the NHS, in churning reform, doesn't allow the tacit anchor to develop, then the motor of judgment stalls' (2008, 50).

In the context of this new, atomised approach to learning and assessment, educational supervision has become a vital focal point. While the idea of supervision for postgraduate doctors is not new, the term 'Educational Supervisor' did not appear until the late 1980s. The role of the Educational Supervisor was explored in the reports *Teaching Hospital Doctors and Dentists to Teach* (SCOPME 1994) and *The Doctor as Teacher* (GMC 1999). As the waves of change in postgraduate teaching and learning gathered pace, the role of Educational Supervisor became more formalised.

Potentially, at least, contact with an Educational Supervisor can provide a space where postgraduate doctors are supported in making sense of their own learning and progression. A key aspect of this support, in successful supervision, lies in encouraging postgraduate doctors to identify and make the best of the many opportunities for learning encountered on hospital wards, in clinics, operating theatres, and in other areas of the workplace. And yet, as illustrated in the quote from an experienced clinical supervisor in Anaesthetics that heads this section, many doctors are unaccustomed to, and perhaps uncomfortable with, explicit talk about learning and teaching. Specifically, as de Cossart and Fish (2005) outline, they may not have made or come to enjoy the parallels between clinical investigation or diagnosis, and the assessment of learning. Yet this type of curiosity may be both transferable and invaluable in the context of educational supervision, raising it far above the level of mechanistic assessment, checking, and form-filling.

PGME has always required doctors to learn in 'service' settings such as hospital wards, clinics, theatres, or laboratories. Further, postgraduate doctors are encouraged to spend time reflecting, for their portfolios contain space for written reflection, and these blank pages are framed as opportunities to admit to uncertainties and to learn from the situations encountered in clinical settings. Yet postgraduate doctors' responses are often brief and far from reflective. Some do not value written reflection; others seem unsure of how to go about this type of learning, which they identify as different to that which they have experienced as medical students. In a recent series of case studies in LEPs, carried out to evaluate QESP, a Foundation Programme [Foundation] Year Two [F2] postgraduate doctor commented:

> I guess the difficulty is differentiating what is teaching and learning, and curriculum, from service.

> I get really interesting feedback from them [Educational Supervisors]. I think that's so much more useful than just going on-line and ticking the

boxes. I mean there's no way that's teaching you much. It's really nice having somebody right there, and the conversation is much more complicated when you're speaking . . . and it's very good to have feedback in words, it's much more real.

I think helping them to give more priority for teaching might improve life for the postgraduate doctors . . . because that's been my biggest bugbear . . . it's all very well having people who are kind of encouraging. But there's limited opportunities for them to directly be teaching.

Here the postgraduate doctor clearly appreciated her one-to-one contact with her Educational Supervisor. She understood the value of conversation about practice, and saw this as educational. Yet she still longed for more 'teaching', making a distinction between 'education' and 'service'. QESP seeks to help both consultants and postgraduate doctors to move from a focus on specific, formal teaching towards a more pervasive interest in the learning opportunities that are to be found everywhere in clinical settings. A reflexive interest in the process of learning itself takes this approach a step further. This may result in positive effects on learners' progress and specifically on exam performance, as Abercombie (1969) suggests in a study of the effects of encouraging medical students to observe, discuss, and reflect on their own reasoning.

## Reflexivity: Putting the Pieces Back Together

I shall move on to explore some of the 'learning stories' from Educational Supervisors and postgraduate doctors that I have encountered in PGME. I shall look at reflexive narrative as one way in which both postgraduate doctors and Educational Supervisors may be encouraged to own and enjoy their learning more fully, to notice learning opportunities, and to locate the necessary propositional learning within the development of wider areas of professional judgement and ethical practice, that is, to develop 'practical wisdom'. As part of this exploration, I will examine what might be learned from the stories of postgraduate doctors whose PGME took place before the national report on *Modernising Medical Careers* (2005), and how their stories might illuminate contemporary PGME. I shall ask what might be revealed about Educational Supervisors' own difficulties and strengths and how their stories might help current postgraduate doctors to understand and articulate their own learning.

At first glance, the structures within which educational supervision takes place might seem inimical to the idea of 'story-telling'. Educational Supervisors may see the postgraduate doctors whom they supervise on only a few occasions – a minimum of three times per rotation (or year) is suggested in the KSS region for Foundation doctors, although, in practice, this varies quite widely, depending on specialty, local arrangements and geographical considerations.

In effect, these structures can make it hard for postgraduate doctors and their Educational Supervisors to establish the kinds of close, supportive and, at the same time, challenging and stimulating professional relationships needed to ensure the best possible progress. These relationships have to be set up quickly, and often seem to be over very quickly, too. Consultants I have worked with have spoken of their frustration at the way in which combinations of annual leave, study leave, and the shorter working hours brought in by the European Working Time Regulations [EWTR] make it hard to get to know their postgraduate doctors well or to assess their understanding and progress in a meaningful way. This is where many feel the loss of the old 'firm' structure most keenly. While the new system's collage of different placements and different experiences may offer postgraduate doctors something of a wide-angle view on PGME, an informed understanding of the career choices open to them, and a chance to test some of these for themselves, many consultants see a downside. The danger is that a postgraduate doctor's development is fragmented: just as their teachers are beginning to understand and attend to their learning needs the postgraduate doctor is whisked away to reinvent the wheel elsewhere, perhaps losing important emerging insights en route.

Educational supervision is, however, a key component in the new system of PGME. Although meetings may be infrequent, they do span a reasonable period of time – typically at least a year for a Foundation doctor. Here there are possibilities similar to those afforded by the one-to-one meetings and professional conversations in QESP (explained further in Chapter 4). Through intense conversation based on the postgraduate doctor's recent practical experience, new understandings can be co-constructed. There is a chance to re-establish coherence in a new way, whereby it is the responsibility of postgraduate doctors to make sense of their own learning. Here, with the Educational Supervisor's support and guidance, postgraduate doctors are able to weigh up the impressions and experiences they have encountered, as well as to consider and follow up on the ideas and skills they need to make their own. They may perhaps also find a space for the emotional and holistic aspects of learning, which can neither be assessed nor denied. As Kathy Feest from the Severn Deanery has put it, 'the lessons of humanity are located in the particular' (Feest 2009, 95).

Supervision meetings can sometimes feel pressured and constrained by the routine tasks that need to be completed: Personal Development Plans, workplace-based assessments, exam preparation, involvement in audits, study leave, attendance on taught programmes, involvement in shifts and other 'service' matters. All of these may jostle for attention during the hour or less set aside for a supervision meeting. Of course, each of these areas in itself can provoke valuable reflection, but under pressure of time it may feel important to 'get all the boxes ticked', leaving little space for exploratory conversation. The learning can remain dry and superficial, unassimilated on deeper levels, such as those relating to the postgraduate doctor's growth as a moral human being and as a professional. Portfolios do require reflective writing, but this too may be completed dutifully with little, if any, sense of the potential value of this activity. Postgraduate doctors doubtless have an eye on their public visibility and the need to be seen to be coping successfully at all times. In narrative terms, this may often seem to necessitate a brief 'victory story' to sum up questions resolved and learning successfully achieved.

A 2002 research project at Emory University in the USA investigated the effects of encouraging 'housestaff' or 'residents' (the equivalent of Foundation and early Specialty postgraduate doctors in the UK) to write narrative accounts of self-selected experiences during the first three years of their postgraduate, hospital-based training (Brady et al 2002). These accounts were kept separate from the residency curriculum, and so were not linked to assessment. Findings suggested that these postgraduate doctors' stories underwent fairly consistent changes, moving from narratives with a focus on 'a search for identity and core values', through a 'period of transition' into 'disillusionment and despair', and in the third year moved towards 'hope and reconciliation'. The patterns, while remaining tentative in this small-scale project, seem to track a process of transformation as the postgraduate doctors underwent an initiation into their lives as clinicians. Interestingly, as in Abercrombie's (1969) research, the authors also concluded that the act of composing these narrative accounts was in itself beneficial in allowing the postgraduate doctors to tell and thereby to start to understand better the stories of their own learning processes:

> Their writings have a spontaneity and genuine honesty that captivate the reader. Such narratives provided us with an understanding of the interplay between the residents' interactions with patients, their own personal issues, and their struggles during several discrete stages of their professional development . . . We believe that such a practice can . . . allow residents to realise that they bring their whole selves – their physical beings, their emotions, their strengths and weaknesses – into each encounter (Brady et al 2002, 220).

In the UK and in the context of educational supervision, oral narrative, the telling of stories, may be a way in which consultants and postgraduate doctors can 'embody' complex understandings, and bring to life abstract or tacit knowledge, while affording value to tentative and exploratory thinking, and resisting the fragmentation of learning that can occur subsequent to the Modernising Medical Careers [MMC] initiative.

The examples of stories that follow were collected with the intention of exploring further the specific characteristics and usefulness of what I am calling 'learning stories' – stories that move away from 'what I learned' to focus on 'how I experienced learning', either systematically or serendipitously. I was interested to find out whether, as in the American case (Brady et al 2002), the act of reflection on and conversation about learning might uncover ideas about learning not included in today's curricula and provide useful evidence of the complex nature of professional learning.

## Four Doctors' Learning Stories

There follow extracts from interviews with three consultants and a final year Specialty Registrar [SpR] working within different specialties in KSS. I have changed their names in order to preserve anonymity. With each interviewee, I recorded and transcribed a conversation of about thirty to forty minutes, and selected extracts to illustrate what I thought were the main themes. In the spirit of qualitative research, I also examined the most interesting less prevalent themes or 'deviant cases' (Green and Thorogood 2008). I acknowledge that my interventions in selecting and shaping these accounts may have moved the extracts I quote away from the speakers' original intentions. At certain points in the conversations, the interviewees presented their memories in the form of longer narratives, which I discuss in more depth in Chapter 6, as I think they contain insights beyond the specific points I set out to illustrate.

Mira is an SpR in Geriatrics, Holly is a consultant geriatrician, James is a consultant in Pain Control, and Harriet is a consultant radiologist.

All three consultants' stories revealed understandably mixed feelings about the changes since MMC. Holly commented positively that 'there is more structured supervision of training, there is curriculum', but was concerned about a lack of continuity:

> At the moment . . . it's more specialty focused and ward based, and the juniors do shifts and they might not follow the patient through. I don't think they see the whole journey.

James's contribution suggests a similar ambivalence:

> I can't honestly remember a single teaching session from my time at a teaching hospital, I did try to think of it but I honestly can't.

> The most valuable thing was the time . . . it didn't feel good at the time, but I had a lot of time with a lot of fantastic clinicians . . . to see a lot of different ways and approaches, and a lot of great, caring people working.

Harriet, too, was ambivalent about the changes, expressing something of the camaraderie inherent in the old-style 'baptism of fire' that doctors expected and often experienced in her day:

> I think the most valuable thing was the team structure and was the hours actually. And the least helpful was the long hours . . . you are dealing with things at the limits, sometimes, of your competence . . . It was a rite of passage that we all had to go through – the long hours, nightmare patients and difficulties – before we could feel we were becoming 'proper doctors'.

The unresolved loss of these rites of passage permeates the consultants' stories, and poses difficult questions in relation to current developments in PGME, questions perhaps not answerable within the terms in which PGME is now formulated.

Each of the doctors talked about relationships between theory and practice, and the ways in which postgraduate doctors' thinking about these develops. Throughout our conversation, Holly described her postgraduate learning as an SpR in terms of 'making real' the ideas and facts she had absorbed during her earlier education and training, explaining that, at this stage, 'it became more clinically relevant'. She characterised this learning as a time of realisation of the complex relationships between theory and practice:

> I tried to start linking it to cases and really realised what all this means. And what does it mean to the patient . . . and how are we going to communicate that with a patient?

Harriet linked these changes to an increased focus on the broader and more integrated aspects of learning to be a doctor. She described how her understanding of learning changed after leaving medical school:

> Being a doctor's not just holding that sort of propositional knowledge . . . It's not just about the theory, it's about the practice, it's about the professionalism, it's about displaying some of the judgement-making skills, integrating it with clinical skills. For me personally it was more about the application of what I had learned. You know, leading up to the finals it was all about learning to pass to be a doctor. But after I had qualified as a doctor it was actually learning the skills that I'd use and employ as a doctor, and making them work for me, and applying them to different people, different settings, different situations, integrating different pieces of knowledge; if something didn't work, what was I going to do about it?

Interestingly, Mira described a more troubled relationship between theory and practice, with memories of some of the fractures that may occur in the transfer between university and practice-based learning:

> I think for me, in my postgraduate training I learned practice first and then I had to go back and almost find a theory when I started teaching more . . . so I just felt like I learned things through hearsay or through trial and error, or people saying 'well this is the way you do this' and just doing it . . . just doing things without knowing why we're doing them really . . . so if I was treating someone with heart failure then I'd put them on an infusion of whatever drug . . . without really thinking through 'Why am I doing this? What's the theoretical basis?'

> When you're a junior you're so busy on the job . . . just trying to get through the day and keep the patients alive . . . you don't have time to go back to theory or books. I'd remember reading things about improving your practice and things like that, and that would just annoy me because I would think I don't have time for improving my practice, I'm just trying to get through.

All three consultants described their learning as a process of self discovery. Harriet's learning story starts with an understanding of her own unique learning style and the ways in which her school experiences influenced and helped to form this:

> I didn't really have too many issues with the clinical, inter-personal aspect, the communication aspect, but I found exams extremely stressful, very anxiety-provoking and difficult hurdles. But that's a personal thing that I've had throughout my life . . . I think it goes back to my own schooling and how I was educated . . . a single-sex school, very strict, very difficult environment . . . and you take that forward with you when you become an adult learner.

In contrast, she found workplace-based learning very well suited to her learning needs, and finds it more useful when it comes to assessing her own postgraduate doctors:

> One of the ways we assess them is, it's not purely on written exams . . . they're able to show their strengths in different areas and I think the current exams seem to be far better at assessing students' overall abilities . . . Now, they do look at how people talk to patients, they do look at how they communicate, and people are assessed on that.

Mira reported a similar preference, one that I imagine to be quite difficult for any hospital doctor to admit to:

> I find that evidence-based practice I really have to work at, and try and make that relevant to me somehow, and reading general science just for science's sake, again I find that very difficult, that doesn't really stick in my head, but if something is going to affect a particular patient today, then that's easy for me to remember and that makes sense to me.

Holly particularly valued one consultant colleague's ability to explicitly share some of his own experiences, commenting that 'these are the things that you're not going to learn in books . . . these are the things that you might encounter'. She added that some of the hardest aspects of her own learning on the way to becoming a consultant were about developing confidence in making relationships – with patients, doctors, nurses – and in making the most of these.

The importance of 'learning about relationships' is identified throughout the consultants' stories as a central aspect of 'making the learning real'. As James comments: 'Nobody ever prepared me for trying to deal with my consultant colleagues'. Holly, too, suggests that the new curricula, whilst paying some attention to communication skills, do not reflect anything like the complexity of a doctor's daily working life:

> Let's start with the tough bits. I think the clinical aspect of the learning . . . I've always enjoyed . . . it's always been quite fascinating and interesting. The tough bits have been . . . dealing with some of the interactions . . . be it with peers or senior colleagues, or even perhaps other health professionals, and perhaps sometimes resolving conflicts which might not have been necessarily clinically related . . . the non-theoretical part of medicine and the day-to-day practice.

Holly's comments also suggested an awareness of the psycho-social aspects of her learning. She suggests a link between 'dealing with human beings on a day-to-day basis' and developing an understanding of hospital hierarchies and management issues. In her own learning story, she identifies the helpful teaching of a particular consultant, who encouraged her at SpR level to find out more about this:

> These aspects are probably not particularly looked at at the moment in the curriculum . . . and until you are actually in the job, the experience is not quite the same . . . He was very keen that at SpR level we get involved in committee meetings . . . and just really observe the interaction . . . [and these were] very good learning experiences.

This had increased her awareness of the complexities of communication within a multi-professional clinical setting, working out who to refer to, for instance, in order to make sure that all aspects of a clinical decision are considered – 'inventing a hierarchy of necessity'.

Holly later described her own further learning through experience she has gained in discovering ways to get the best out of the teams and colleagues she works with – 'valuing the team members':

> When we do something well everybody gets a credit, not just the consultant or the doctors . . . so for example when I get a thank-you letter I make sure that all the ward know about it, so nurses know and we take a copy onto the ward.

She linked the idea of respect to her increasing confidence in giving useful and honest feedback:

> I think I know how to handle the situation . . . to point out that there was an issue there . . . but for them to look on it as an experience . . . because sometimes the postgraduate doctor could end up blaming themself and that could be quite a negative experience . . . It's very subtle. For example, there was a communication problem and it led to this person being upset or led to a problem with prescribing something . . . but how are we going to help the postgraduate doctor to learn through it?

An understanding that professional 'education', as opposed to 'training', involves and changes the whole person, is implicit in these stories. One of the ways in which Holly says she feels that she has matured as a professional is in bringing her own wider human experience to bear on her professional practice. For instance, she saw connections between her own experience of illness within the family, and the understanding she hopes to encourage in her current postgraduate doctors:

> [During my mother's illness] I was still a professional and I was still expected to know all the medical signs and complications and what chemotherapy does . . . but I was also a worried, stressed, very concerned daughter . . .

trying to speak to someone about what's happening today, and I wasn't getting through because they were doing a ward-round. Maybe the positive outcome of it is actually I do appreciate when people phone and are wanting [to know more] . . . I try to say to the team members it is actually quite difficult to be in that situation, and you have to appreciate that.

In the following chapter, I explore more extended 'learning stories' told by the same group of consultants, in order to pursue further aspects of their holistic learning. Those stories and the ideas expressed here represent and illustrate, I think, deeply held convictions on the part of the doctors I interviewed. And yet these realisations are not on the official map of postgraduate doctors' learning. Such stories illuminate the process of assimilating all the complex and often tacit information that a postgraduate doctor needs to acquire in some way if they are to succeed in becoming a good doctor. I return to the question posed at the start of this chapter: do stories have a place in educational supervision? With all the pressures and calls on their time and attention, many Educational Supervisors will feel that such a practice, if it ever existed, has been driven out by the new competence-led NCFs. And yet, despite these difficulties, in many of the meetings I have observed during my work as an ADE, Educational Supervisors have managed to find ways to work with postgraduate doctors on this important developmental level. Sometimes simply by asking open but informed questions, and then listening intently, they have elicited narratives that move the conversation into a more reflective mode – into the 'third space', as discussed by Rachel Robinson in Chapter 4. Here postgraduate doctors explore and strengthen their ability to locate, articulate and extend the learning that occurs during clinical practice.

A reflexive approach implies taking this even further, to the point where the postgraduate doctor is able to learn something about learning itself, through consideration of their own contexts, constraints, and progress. Thus, educational supervision is inextricable from, and a vital aspect of, postgraduate teaching and learning in clinical settings. Where educational supervision works well, it allows for a form of professional conversation, in which postgraduate doctors make links between their theoretical learning and the more subtle aspects of clinical and professional practice – locating 'episteme' within 'gnosis' (see Chapter 2) – by relating those forms of learning to their own specific learning stories. At the same time, adding to the complexity of these interactions are the conventions of traditional narrative form. The learner may need to resist the narrative conventions that insist on a rapid progression from problem through complication towards resolution. In some professional conversations, there is an almost tangible sense of the postgraduate doctor's increasing ability to sustain moments of uncertainty, resisting 'closure' on a case or issue, in order to think further.

As an example, the following extract is taken from a consultant's written reflections after a QESP professional conversation. This very experienced consultant psychiatrist was delighted with the results of a shift of emphasis, whereby she had started to encourage her General Practice postgraduate doctor to describe recent experiences and to discuss his own learning, rather than her simply 'feeding back' to him her assessment of his work. The postgraduate doctor brought to the session a story in which he felt he was beginning to gain confidence in history taking, something he had struggled with in the past. His patient, who had been discovered wandering in an abandoned area of the local docklands, was well known to the hospital. Thus, the learner might be expected to move very quickly from problem to resolution, relying on a pre-existing narrative. However, through careful listening he had been able to resist that closure, and instead to respond with a level of intuition that had previously eluded him. He was thus able to come up with new ideas in relation to this patient's case:

> He was able to reflect on what he's learned in an insightful way . . . He mentioned how he did not find the pro formas helpful in assessing clients and was taking history in more depth. This showed that he was able to get the message I had been trying to convey through joint assessments and discussions in an indirect way. He approached people as individuals and tried to understand their problems rather than tick boxes, without losing the goal of reaching some degree of formulation to guide in planning the management.

This confident uncertainty seems to me to be a significant sign of progress into professional competence. The use of narrative is one powerful way in which such progress may be supported.

## Outside the Boxes

Stories such as those collected here say a great deal about what lies beyond the ticking of boxes, and can spark useful thinking. Clearly, there is limited time available for doctors to meet and engage in such reflective and reflexive practice, and yet without it the practice of educational supervision can be a dry and unrewarding experience, and poor use of precious time. However, in this respect, a little goes a long way. It is not possible to 'cover' everything – and, in fact, a narrative approach may be especially helpful in this context. One fulfilling experience of shared reflective practice around a specific learning story may enable both postgraduate doctor and supervisor to think more fully at other times, on less formal occasions. It may enable a more resourceful, more sure-footed and critical kind of meaning-making as doctors' learning stories continue to evolve.

# References

Abercrombie, M. L. J. 1969. *The Anatomy of Judgement*. London: Pelican.

Brady, D. W., G. Corbie-Smith, and W. T. Branch Jr. 2002. "What's important to you?": The use of narratives to promote self-reflection and to understand the experiences of medical residents. *Annals of Internal Medicine*, 137(3), 220-223.

Feest, K. 2009. Introducing Narrative Reflection. *Essential Guide to Educational Supervision in Postgraduate Medical Education*. eds. Cooper, N. and K. Forrest, 2009. Chichester: Wiley-Blackwell/ BMJ Books

de Cossart, L. and D. Fish. 2005. *Cultivating a Thinking Surgeon*. Shrewsbury: tfm Publishing Ltd.

Fish, D. and L. de Cossart. 2007. *Developing the Wise Doctor*. London: Royal Society of Medicine Press.

*The Doctor as Teacher*. 1990. London: General Medical Council.

Green, J. and N. Thorogood. 2008. *Qualitative Methods for Health Research*. London: Sage.

Sennett, R. 2008. *The Craftsman*. London: Allen Lane.

*Teaching Hospital Doctors and Dentists to Teach*. 1994. London: SCOPME.

Vygotsky, L. 1962. *Thought and Language*. London: MIT Press.

# Seven Learning Stories

I have collected seven slightly longer stories from the group of consultants whose contributions are discussed in Chapter 5. These raise more complex and interwoven ideas about learning in clinical settings. I have commented on each from my own perspective as an educationist, but I am, of course, aware that they may suggest different readings to other readers and, in particular, to clinicians. These stories and the ways in which they have been narrated may have a familiar ring. They could be seen as archetypal, illustrating some of the ways in which doctors commonly understand their world and their induction into it. In this sense the stories may offer insights into doctors' learning, how they understood it, and the assumptions and values that underlie their understandings.

## Stories and Narratives

These oral accounts were tape-recorded during interviews and later transcribed. In each interview, after some initial general talk, I asked brief open questions in order to elicit longer responses. The questions had been sent out in advance to allow each doctor a chance to think about their learning stories, and to call to mind instances which they identified as important to their development.

In my commentaries, I refer both to *stories* and to *narratives*. These words are often used interchangeably. By *story*, I mean the sequence of events related by each of the tellers. *Narrative* refers to the way of telling – the particular expression of the story by its narrator, its ordering or structure, and the language and imagery used. Interestingly, the word 'narrative' derives from the Proto-Indo-European root 'gno-', meaning 'to know'. It is, therefore, closely related to 'gnosis' (see Chapter 2). Narrative is a way of knowing. It can express the integrated understanding that develops over time. It is, moreover, impossible to contain within a tick-box. I have mainly referred to these accounts as stories, but in some cases my commentary has focused on aspects of the narrative.

The work of Arthur W Frank of the University of Calgary may also be of relevance in considering these stories. Frank has written on the 'illness narratives' told by patients. He categorises these narratives into three main types: 'restitution', 'chaos', and 'quest' (Frank 1995). He suggests that, in the West we tend to seek restitution narratives, in which the patient is first well, then becomes ill, and finally regains their health. In a chaos narrative, there is no such coherence or recovery; Frank characterises such accounts as 'anti-narratives'. Quest narrative presents a patient's illness and suffering as a journey, in which something may be gained from the experience through exploration and, possibly, through a reinterpretation of illness itself. Clearly, the stories told by patients will be very different to those told by doctors. However, I feel that the characteristics of Frank's narrative types are paralleled in the experiences related by doctors below. Western medicine offers us all the promise of restitution, and some of these stories hinge on the difficulties faced by doctors in trying to provide this.

## Story One: Mira
## Beyond the Guidelines

Mira's story of a difficult early experience with a terminally ill patient reveals an aspect of learning about the difficulty of working to guidelines. Faced with the unexpected necessity to 'break bad news' to a patient, she found herself unable to resist offering some form of restitution:

> I had a patient, she was probably in her late thirties and she had melanoma that had spread, and she was obviously dying, she'd come to the end of chemo, there was nothing more they could do for her. I was talking to her and her husband . . . I think I was just on a normal morning ward-round . . . and somehow it came up, this thing about being resuscitated . . . And she said 'What! You're not going to resuscitate me?' and was completely shocked by that fact. And I was shocked that that she was shocked, and it was a bit of a difficult situation really. I wasn't sure what to do. So I said 'Well yes, no that's fine, if you want to be for resuscitation then of course we'll keep you for resus', you know, 'it's your choice' sort of thing. Now I teach, or try to teach guidelines for making these decisions, and I've realised that it wasn't her choice at all, it was a clinical decision, and if you say that you're not going to, that resuscitation is not the right treatment for a patient, you don't have to do it. But at the time, that didn't feel like the right thing to do, and so I guess what I do with the students is I use that as an example. Sometimes you totally break the guidelines just because it feels too wrong to say to a thirty-something-year-old 'no I'm not going to resuscitate you because it wouldn't be right'.

On TV there's this idea that you resuscitate someone and then they sit up and say 'thank you very much doc.' But real life is that most resuscitation attempts fail . . . if someone is dying . . . then attempts to resuscitate them wouldn't work, and therefore it becomes a very undignified way to die, with a whole team of people jumping up and down on your chest, trying to give you shots, trying to bring you back. When actually it would be much more dignified to have a morphine drip to give you pain relief, and your family holding your hand. That was probably the conversation I should have had with her at the time. If I was seeing that patient now, as a more experienced doctor, I'd be able to have that conversation with her and explain it all much more clearly, but at that time I just didn't know, I was young and hadn't done much in the way of having life-affecting decision conversations.

In this very honest account, Mira shows how hard it can be for an inexperienced doctor to find the right words. The patient's shock precipitates her own shock and confusion, and there seems to be no right way out of the situation, no story to tell that could possibly get things back on the right track. She perceives the TV story of the heroic doctor as another narrative standing in the way of more helpful communication with the patient and her husband: there ought to be something that she, as the doctor, can do to save this young woman's life. Conflicting values add further complexity. Mira's desire to do what is right, to respect the patient's wishes, to offer her a story that would seem more appropriate for such a young patient, conflicts with the need to follow protocol, and with Mira's theoretical understanding that attempted resuscitation would not produce a good outcome for her patient.

There is a good illustration here, I believe, of the danger that a protocol, while purporting to solve a problem or to make a decision easy or inevitable, may suddenly seem inadequate in the face of an unpredictable situation, a real patient, real suffering. I feel that Mira's use of this story with her own students is particularly admirable. She is open about her own early uncertainties, allowing the students the opportunity to admit to theirs. She rehearses for them the moment when they have to apply what they know, opening the way to discussion of the difficulties they may encounter. She comments 'now I teach, or try to teach guidelines'. The phrase 'try to teach' demonstrates her understanding of the tenuous and difficult nature of this learning. It is very far from being a simple matter of transmission of information.

## Story Two: Holly
## Learning from a Patient with Cancer

Holly's story about learning from a patient also focuses on 'breaking bad news', an area of communication that receives particular attention during postgraduate medical education [PGME]. In this instance, a subtle and surprising relationship starts to develop between a new consultant and a terminally ill physics professor:

I can give you an experience . . . [where] I think actually I learned from the patient. I had just been appointed as a consultant, and there was a professor of physics and he was diagnosed with cancer and it was a very, very emotional time for everyone . . . He was highly intelligent, and he wanted to know, so I had to tell him what's going on. Then I had to have this meeting with him and his daughter, and . . . breaking the news in a more official way to him, although he already had some understanding, and there was a very difficult situation.

But in fact it was interesting, because when he realised I was finding it difficult to get the message across to the daughter, the patient then almost took over . . . And so he started by asking 'Okay, how long have I got?' . . . because he said 'I need to plan this and that' . . . and in the end I tried to round it up to say 'Actually I know that must be a very difficult situation for the family', and I said 'It's actually quite difficult for us to break bad news, and it doesn't get any easier, regardless of what level we are'.

And the fascinating thing is that he said to me, and I must say I felt I didn't handle that situation maybe as well as it could have been, but he actually said to me 'And you did that very well'. I think I acknowledged that as a difficult situation . . . and I was trying to be very open and understanding of the situation . . . and I think there was a lot of honesty in it.

This story stands in its own right, and will, of course, yield different meanings for different readers. In my own reading, I found myself particularly interested in what it shows about the intricate play between learning and teaching in any professional's development. Here Holly is both a teacher, when attempting to help the family to come to terms with the patient's prognosis, while at the same time she is also a learner, who is vulnerable in the face of the task she has to perform, and who benefits from her patient's 'practical wisdom'.

## Story Three: Harriet
## Half an Hour's Sleep

This is a full version of Harriet's story about 'initiation', as mentioned briefly in Chapter 5. It is a story I have heard told in many ways and on many occasions by doctors worried about the changes in PGME. Harriet's version deals with the double-edged nature of long hours and a culture that required her to be seen as suffering to gain professional recognition. She experienced this as the worst and also the best of times:

I think the most valuable thing was the team structure and was the hours actually. And the least helpful was the long hours. And it's a very difficult thing, because I can remember as a houseman my on-call . . . my weekend duty, I did a one in three, I think, for one of my jobs, so I was on call every third night, and I can remember it starting at nine o'clock on a Friday morning, you could attend an optional ward-round at eight, but it started at nine, and it finished at five o'clock on Monday. And I was working and available for work for the entire time. Now that was exhausting, absolutely exhausting, but I think some of the most sort of incredible learning opportunities happened over that time, whether they were clinical, personal . . .

I think you learn a lot about yourself, your abilities and limitations, and that inevitably leads to insight. And you are dealing with things at the limits, sometimes, of your competence . . . But the very strict team structure meant that whatever decisions you made, you had to take responsibility and you had to account for those decisions, whether they were right or wrong. So the ward-round the following day always meant that you could be ridiculed or lambasted or told you'd done a great job and saved somebody's life . . . or just everything was okay.

There was a huge 'Oh, my on-call was really busy, I got half an hour's sleep!' 'Well mine was even busier and we admitted forty patients!' And there's a lot of that metaphorical 'mine's bigger than yours!' So I think it was part of it, you had to put your hours in, in order to achieve the level of being a doctor that you wanted to achieve. It was a rite of passage that we all had to go through – the long hours, nightmare patients and difficulties – before we could feel we were becoming 'proper doctors' . . . now without these extended hours, what has taken place for the newer breed? How do they earn their badges? Do they feel they are 'proper doctors' if they have never seen many of the conditions we encountered?

Harriet's assertion that, in her day you learned 'insight' through working at 'the limits of your competence' may help to explain an ambivalence that she and others feel about the new generation of learning stories. Shorter working hours mean that postgraduate doctors may not see so many conditions, and this may affect their levels of confidence and competence. But what comes across much more strongly here is Harriet's memory of this time as a 'rite of passage', a quest undertaken alone into the almost unknown, fraught with danger. The final sense of camaraderie and exhilaration is here described as inextricable from the exhaustion and possible humiliation, if anything should have gone wrong. This story conjures up ideas of adventure, competition, striving, and conquest. There is the sense that these experiences, while related with some irony, were truly transformative. And 'insight' is very highly valued by the clinicians I have worked with. A doctor lacking insight may be viewed as a hopeless case, and insight is often said to be a quality almost impossible to teach.

This quest narrative, in which the postgraduate doctor squeezes through the eye of the needle at great personal risk, could be seen to represent metaphorically the idea that the learner must in some way strike out on their own if they are to become a 'proper doctor'. Today, this independence is formulated more in terms of the postgraduate doctor's responsibility to keep and develop a portfolio, and to seek out opportunities for learning through workplace-based assessments – a quieter and far less heroic version of the quest for professional competence. Consultants like Harriet are prepared to work in new, more humanistic ways with postgraduate doctors, acknowledging that their past experiences of having to work 'at the limits' were in some ways 'the least helpful' aspect of their learning. Although PGME has changed considerably, therefore, this type of story still exerts a powerful influence and should perhaps be acknowledged as a determining factor in the ways in which contemporary postgraduate doctors are viewed and judged.

## Story Four: James
## Heroes and Mentors

James's stories also suggest the idea of a quest, since they focus on overcoming difficulties through taking initiative. He describes the way in which he, in effect, invented his own career pathway at a formative time for his particular specialty. He is, however, quick to acknowledge the guidance that came his way, despite the winding path of his learning. His story illustrates the qualities and benefits of the informal teaching and mentoring he received. His most striking role models were clinicians who were able and willing to admit their own mistakes and uncertainties, and who insisted on the importance of a principled approach and of being open to learning from patients:

> There was a chap . . . who was very good . . . very encouraging and helpful, and he would organise anything. He would always say he didn't really know, though he was a very knowledgeable chap . . . I still practise very much the way I learned from him . . . I think it was all sort of tacit, it was working with him, watching how he dealt with patients . . . He was hugely against this idea that we should have our own likes or dislikes or our own ideas about what the right treatment is, there was a patient there and you had to find what was right for the patient . . . as opposed to what was right for science, or for the department.

> The chap who started me in Anaesthetics . . . was brilliant because he'd sit there, he'd light up a cigarette and if something was forthcoming we would talk about it, or if something had been planned, but if not, as like as not, he'd say 'Oh dear, now I've made a terrible mess of this' or 'That really was very close there'. It worked on a number of levels because not only did it encourage you to be honest about your mistakes and things you'd done wrong, things you hadn't thought out properly. It encouraged us to open up and discuss . . . he always said it was actually us talking amongst ourselves that was the best bit. There was a lot of discussion, I can remember, and . . . even people who didn't find it easy to talk in groups . . . after a while would become quite open and admit to the same hassles and difficulties as the rest of us.

James clearly benefited from another doctor's mature ability to admit to, and learn from, mistakes. His account also describes a rare kind of spaciousness that he was fortunate enough to experience in the extremely busy world of a hospital: the idea that his mentor would 'sit there and light up a cigarette' (placing this narrative very clearly in the past!), and allow the postgraduate doctors to take their time, so that 'after a while' they would 'become quite open'. Again, ambivalent feelings about the past surface in this account. Postgraduate doctors were previously placed under extreme pressure and largely expected to find their own way (James had earlier commented on the lack of formal teaching when he was in training). Yet there was a sense of community and a 'mess', a location away from the wards where conversations could take place in a more relaxed way. There was also a career structure (or lack of structure) which allowed for individual variation in terms of the time taken to arrive at consultant grade.

## Story Five: Harriet
## He Nearly Died

Of course, most doctors have 'near miss' stories, moments of personal or organisational error, or sheer bad luck, which form unforgettable learning memories. These may well arise in the kinds of stressful situations described in Harriet's previous account (Story Three). In this second story from Harriet she expands on this idea, identifying her learning as both clinical and inter-professional:

> I still remember certain things that happened and relate them to certain patients I saw fifteen years ago.

> Often my learning experiences happened when I was on call or on a night duty in an A&E . . . They happened outside of normal working hours, in fact all of them have. The key thing is that I remember, because I think they all taught me a lot about myself, a lot about how I operate under stress or in difficult situations, they taught me a lot about the people I worked with, as well as various conditions . . .

> One was a young man who was stabbed in North London, I can remember saying to the nurse, you know, 'it's a tiny wound' and she was a sort of a big, Irish casualty staff nurse who more or less said to me 'you know, you may be the doctor, I've got years of experience however and I'll tell you that young man is sick'. And I didn't really take on board what she was saying ... It's a very powerful word because you say, you know, 'well or sick' or 'well or ill', and stand at the end of the bed, look at somebody and it's the snap gut feeling, they're ill, they're well, they're okay, we can leave them for a bit, and I suppose I hadn't really listened to her and I hadn't taken it on board ... And sure enough the guy crashed and ... there was something like a nine-inch blade that had gone through and cut his liver and through his stomach up into his chest ... That was another sort of moment, partly because the

patient nearly died, where I thought 'actually, you know, I may be a doctor but she's far better than me'. She was more experienced, even though she was a nurse, she had the experience, which I didn't have. And that sort of made me very respectful and very mindful of other people's experience. And listening to them, you know, clinical work is often about teamwork.

There are many interesting threads in this narrative. Harriet, like Mira, displays great humility. There is a sense in which her story is told against the grain. In her previous story she mentions the 'ridicule' and 'lambasting' that might well result from the exposure of a poor clinical judgement. Making mistakes was, and still is, both a necessary facet of learning, and also extremely difficult to admit to in clinical settings. It is not that the inevitability of human error is unacknowledged in medicine. Surgeon Atul Gawande, for instance, has written extensively on this in his books *Complications* (2003) and *Better* (2008). Gawande comments: 'In surgery, as in anything else, skill and confidence are learned through experience – haltingly and humiliatingly . . . There is one difference in medicine, though; it is people we practice upon' (2003,18).

Doctors are supposed to have authority on the ward; to learn in this way from a nurse may not be easy. Harriet identifies the 'snap gut feeling' she was trying to develop at this particular stage of her own development, again linking this to 'experience' and, crucially, suggesting the importance of 'listening' to other professionals in order to learn and gain insight.

Another thread that links this to other doctors' stories is the focus on clinicians' use of language. The nurse identifies the patient as 'sick', and Harriet says that she failed at the time to understand this as a 'very powerful word'. In this context, and between clinicians, 'sick' translates as 'very ill indeed'. She is describing a moment in her induction into a highly specific and scrupulous language register.

## Story Six: Harriet
## A Light Bulb Moment

Harriet's story about how she learned to perform a good biopsy suggests an understanding of a clinical version of what Richard Sennett (2008) has termed 'material consciousness'. Sennett (2008, 146) quotes William Carlos Williams's declaration 'that there should be "no ideas but in things"'. Sennett describes a way of knowing that is concerned with 'the link between hand and head' – a link made every day by doctors in their work with human beings and their bodies. This type of learning is very hard to put into words, but Harriet's account comes close:

> Something I'm reasonably good at is biopsying things . . . targeted biopsies . . . which is useful because sometimes it can save people an operation, sometimes it means you find out what's wrong with them with a small procedure, but I can remember somebody showing me how to do it and it

was almost like one of those light bulb moments where I just thought 'Oh of course, that's so obvious', and I think because I am more practical than anything it became, you know . . . I can do it very easily now.

You're basically biopsying a lump somewhere in the body, but that lump can be in something or around something or just there. But I think my particular pleasure, if you like, in doing is that most people come out and say 'That was nowhere near bad as I thought it was going to be', or 'Gosh that was over quick and I thought it was going to be awful' or 'You didn't hurt me at all', all of those things which are, for me, positive outcomes.

I think it's experiential. I think it's reflection on when it doesn't go right, and I think linked into that is an insight into what you can and can't do. I think in part it's a sort of a healthy respect for the body, you know, you have to think quite carefully about where you're going to stick a needle into somebody, so that requires anatomical knowledge and things like that, and then . . .

In the first instance somebody showed me how to do it, and they made it very explicit, I suppose, what I was meant to do and actually almost told me the theory of it in a physical way . . . If you're putting a needle into somebody and you're trying to look at it with an ultrasound beam that's a few millimetres thick . . . how you do it is you need to see the needle going throughout the length so you need to keep this hand still, move this . . .

And what's interesting is then seeing other people try and do it and seeing that actually they've not had the benefit of that. You know? And it just looks all so ham-fisted!

Here, Harriet uses the word 'insight' to try to identify the component in her learning that goes beyond 'healthy respect for the body' and beyond 'anatomical knowledge'. Her teacher 'almost told me the theory of it in a physical way'. The physical skill, reliant on eye, hand, and head, is also inextricable from the values that she expresses in her delight that her patients do not suffer unnecessarily and may be spared an unnecessary procedure, and in her pride in the knowledge that she is able to do this procedure very well.

## Story Seven: Holly
## A Difficult Time

I asked Holly if she had a story of a difficult time in her career, a time when she had felt like giving up. She had spoken so positively about her work and learning that I thought it unlikely that she would have much to say at this point. However, this was her story:

I can think of one incident that happened to me during my training. I was very upset by it, by what happened to the patient. A lady came in very unwell with suspected meningitis, and I did a lumbar puncture, but unfortunately she deteriorated. We contacted neurosurgeons . . . It was a very rare thing to occur after lumbar puncture, but unfortunately she died. She had meningococcal meningitis . . . and then she was quite sick and she might not have survived anyway, [but] I felt very bad about it for quite some time. I started questioning my clinical judgement . . . my competence.

In the immediate first few days, I think I spoke with a number of people, of experts, and I approached the anaesthetist, approached the neurologist, to see would they still have done the lumbar puncture given the same scenario. They were all quite supportive . . . given the same situation they would have done the same. They gave me papers as well, and the papers were saying that you have to be cautious and this and that in this situation, but for me, it was very important to know that my peers would have probably done the same.

I will always remember . . . my consultant was away. And realising what had happened he actually phoned, he was skiing, on holiday, he phoned to see how I felt, and I really appreciated that. He realised what the impact of this would be on me, it meant so much.

Holly's last comment here says a great deal, I think, about the weight of responsibility taken on by any doctor new to this role. In terms of Frank's narrative types, this is a chaos narrative. She describes herself in terms that might just as well apply to a patient's convalescence 'in the immediate first few days'. Casting about for reassurance, she experienced, perhaps more acutely than ever before, what has been described in Chapter 2 as 'tragic guilt'. She had acted as well as she could within the limits of her knowledge and of the information available, but had not been able to save her patient. There was no restitution.

## Staying Alive

Collecting these doctors' learning stories, re-reading and reflecting on them has been an eye-opening experience. Despite the narrators' concerns about the present and future of medicine as a profession, the narratives are full of life. These are vital stories, recalled in detail and with strong feeling. I have been particularly struck and heartened by the commitment to learning, and interest in its complexities that emerged. Learning should be exciting, and this group of learners and teachers convey this very clearly. There is evidence of their appreciation that learning and teaching in clinical settings may work best when least expected or planned for. Events that at the time seemed chaotic, or caused these learners dismay, have later been assimilated as part of the accumulation of learning memories that leads toward competence in clinical decision making and a mature understanding of professionalism.

Returning to the relevance of these stories to clinical and educational supervision, I would argue that there is a place and, in fact, a need for narrative as part of the learning process. Teachers often refer to 'the steps to learning' – the stages through which a learner needs to pass in order to develop a skill or understanding. Most of us find it very difficult to remember these steps: they are like a ladder that we kick away on arrival at the understanding we have been seeking. Effective teachers often seem to have the ability to recall and articulate these stages or steps, so that they are able to 'break down learning' into readily understandable parts or stages. I would argue that the use of narrative is a helpful way in which to gain access to at least some of these stages, and for teachers to accompany learners on their learning journeys. At the very least, it may increase the interest of both teacher and learner in the fascinating complexities of learning.

In my experience as a teacher, it has frequently been necessary to take in new information, new curricula, and new systems of assessment, and it has often been hard or impossible to accept that these will actually improve anything. It can be difficult to keep alive the best of what one already knows, and one's own hard-won insights, while staying open to new practices. In contemporary PGME and the new curricula, there is a danger that the learning is dissected and itemised to such an extent, that educational supervision becomes an arid and reductive activity. Narrative can be a powerful way to keep learning alive.

# References

Frank, A.W. 1995.*The Wounded Storyteller*. Chicago/London: The University of Chicago Press.

Gawande, A. 2003. *Complications*. London: Profile Books Ltd.

Gawande, A. 2008. *Better*. London: Profile Books Ltd.

Sennett, R. 2008. *The Craftsman*. London: Allen Lane.

# Doctor Means Teacher: the Impact of an MA Education in Clinical Settings

Medical doctors perform a dual role in their day-to-day practice in clinical settings. They not only care for, and treat, patients, but they also teach the next generation of doctors, including medical students, and postgraduate doctors. Meeting this commitment to teach undergraduate and postgraduate doctors, alongside, and as part of, their clinical work, is a complex task for doctors; all the more so, because the role of teacher is one for which doctors have traditionally received little formal preparation or ongoing support (Pugsley and McCrorie 2007). Extensive structural change to postgraduate medical education [PGME] in the UK over the last five years has resulted in more attention being paid to the teaching roles that hospital doctors and general practitioners [GPs] perform. There are now increasing numbers of courses (both compulsory and elective) that are aimed at developing doctors as teachers. Yet, the focus of these courses is on the development of effective techniques for use in formal classroom-based teaching, rather than a focus on how to maximise teaching and learning in the real-life clinical context.

Arriving to work in the field of PGME from the broader field of mainstream education, I was rather baffled to see that, outside the Kent, Surrey and Sussex Postgraduate Medical Deanery [KSS], there was considerable emphasis upon 'one-shot workshops', and e-learning modules as the main means of supporting doctors in their work as teachers. My perplexity was that I had entered a field that placed a lot of emphasis on evidence-based practice, and yet there is substantial proof from a well-established body of research on teacher education and professional development, that one-off workshops do not work as well as interventions, to support teachers in deep and sustained development of their practice (see, for instance, Richardson 2003; Stein et al 1999). Rather, the kinds of interventions that support teachers in developing their practice, are long-term programmes, which are predicated on analysing practice 'in situ', and which involve participants working together to engage in structured critical inquiry of their practice (Avalos In press; Borko 2004; Lieberman 1994). Given that doctors teach in a more complex variety of contexts than classroom teachers do, and that they have to juggle their teaching responsibilities alongside their clinical commitments, it seems all the more important for them to be provided with very carefully structured support programmes, in which to develop their teaching practice.

In sum, my observations of doctors working as teachers in clinical settings have engendered two predominant feelings: awe at the commitment many have to the crucial task of educating the next generation of doctors, and concern at the scant support they have traditionally received for this role. In comparison with the rest of the UK, KSS provides substantial support for the teaching role that doctors perform. In the UK, however, the norm has been for doctors to be left largely to their own devices in terms of developing their teaching. For some, this means that they seek out postgraduate programmes focused on clinical education. Most doctors, however, are left to develop their teaching practice 'on the hoof', with perhaps an occasional workshop on teaching thrown in.

I think that there are two main reasons for this trend of expecting doctors to 'get on with the job' of teaching in PGME, with little ongoing structured support. The first is that, until relatively recently, there has been a lack of educational leadership in the field of PGME, and so the formation of educational strategy within hospitals and other clinical settings has been the exception rather than the norm. The second reason is that the field of research into PGME, being a relatively nascent one, tends to make few references to relevant studies and theories in the broader field of educational research (Kogana and Shea 2007; Pugsley and McCrorie 2007). There is, therefore, a dearth of research on the kind of professional development programmes that work to help doctors make meaningful and sustained changes to their practice as teachers.

In this chapter, I seek to respond to the lack of research on the impact of professional development programmes on the teaching practice of doctors. I do so by reporting on a small-scale qualitative study, a central aim of which was to examine the effect of a part-time MA Education in Clinical Settings programme on the practice of the doctors who have completed, or were completing, the course. In total, I interviewed nine participants in semi-structured interviews that were about forty minutes in duration. Eight of the doctors had completed the programme in the last three years, and one was in the final year of the programme. I also analysed exit surveys, completed by a total of fifteen MA students, all of whom completed the programme between 2009 and 2010. The themes I report on in this chapter are informed also by the ongoing informal conversations and communications I have had with MA students and alumni in my role as module leader and past course leader for this programme.

In the following section, I summarise, by way of introduction, the broad structures and purposes of the MA Education in Clinical Settings. I then report on how doctors describe the impact of the programme on their practice. In the final section, I present some implications of this study for the kind of teaching support that is provided for doctors within PGME in the UK, and beyond.

## The Structure of the MA Education in Clinical Settings

The MA Education in Clinical Settings is led and taught by the Education Department at KSS, and validated through the University of Brighton. At any one time, there are between thirty and forty students on the course. Broadly speaking, the course objectives are to provide participants with occasion to engage in structured research on their practice as educators, and thereby to develop both their teaching practice, and a capacity to become educational change agents. Throughout the course, participants are introduced to a range of educational theories on foundational topics such as teaching and learning, practitioner research methods, language study, inter-professional learning, learning in organisations, curriculum, and practitioner research processes.

On the course, participants are required to reflect critically on their own practice as teachers in clinical settings. In this way, the MA course shares a set of common principles with the KSS Qualified Educational Supervisor Programme [QESP], discussed in Chapters 4, 5 and 6. However, a key difference between QESP and the MA Education in Clinical Settings is the way in which the latter aims for participants to 'know thyself' as a teacher, as a foundation to developing as researchers, and as change agents within PGME. Otherwise put, the aims of the MA Education in Clinical Settings are to equip doctors not only to be able to continually develop their own teaching practice, but also to be able to apply relevant research methodologies and educational theory, in order to study and develop teaching practice in their local setting, and thereby to become change agents within a broader educational landscape.

Like me, those who teach on the MA Education in Clinical Settings are educationists, whose previous experience is within mainstream education (including school teaching, teacher education, professional development for teachers, and educational research). As a course team, we all vary slightly in our educational philosophies. Yet, the principled approach to practice described in Chapter 2 is an ethical framework that we share, and one that underpins our approach as teachers on the MA Education in Clinical Settings programme. There are many facets to this ethical framework, and I do not want to reduce it to a set of sound bites. However, I think it is fair to say that our practice as teachers on the MA Education in Clinical Settings rests on three core principles: first, that learning to teach is an ongoing process; second, that teaching is better understood as an art than a science; and third, that the journey to becoming a change agent for educational practice has to be 'inside-out' – that is, beginning with a deep understanding of one's own practice as a teacher and learner.

Given this set of principles embodied within the course team, and the modules that comprise the MA course, it is not at all surprising that what I would term the central narrative or *gestalt* emerging from the set of conversations I had with one student and seven alumni of the MA Education in Clinical Settings, was that the impact of the course is of an ongoing, unfolding variety. As one doctor put it:

> I think it's sort of a constant presence . . . it's not something that I think about all the time, but it's not something I've completely forgotten, but it

is something I go back to all the time (Doctor A).

Doctors described this process of change as one where they gradually became more reflective about their practice, through seeing the complexity of teaching, and where they gradually became aware of the underlying beliefs, values and ideals, which shaped their personal teaching practice, as evidenced in the following comments:

> The course has helped to clarify some of my values and beliefs, and made me think a lot more about the responsibilities of being a teacher and educator. I really think that education should be emancipating and inspiring, and the course has confirmed that (Doctor C).

> [The course] has changed my perspective on learning and education fundamentally, and has opened up avenues and ideas for further work, audits, research. It has also kept me thinking and reflecting on my own and others' teaching (Doctor B).

The doctors above report that the course has caused them to make shifts in their stance as educators. They no longer view teaching as performance, but are beginning to see it as a relational act. In the following sections, I enlarge upon this central narrative; I also explore some of the interesting side roads that were revealed through my conversations with the doctors who have completed the MA Education in Clinical Settings.

## First Steps into the MA: Shock of the New

As a course team, one of the points we make to doctors who evince interest in doing the MA programme is that, although the course is very grounded in a critical analysis of practice, it is not one in which we will be introducing them to 'tips and tricks' for teaching. We say this, not because we believe that there is no such thing as an effective teaching technique. Rather, we say it because learning the techniques of effective teaching is a very small part of the journey of learning to be a good teacher. The much larger part of the journey is the development of one's practical wisdom as a teacher (Sockett 1993, 62). One way of understanding what comprises the practical wisdom of teaching is to see it constellating around three foci: knowledge of self, knowledge of students, and knowledge of subject.

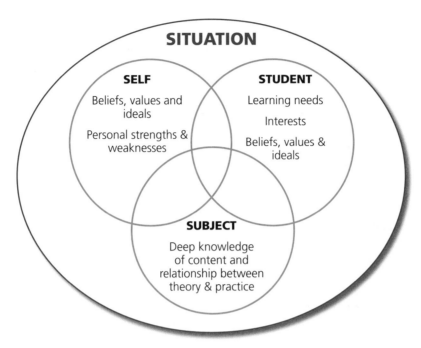

Figure 1: A model of the practical wisdom of teaching

In this model we see three interlinked aspects of the practical wisdom of teaching. The deeper the teacher's knowledge of each element, and of the way it connects to the other elements, the greater the likelihood of pedagogical effectiveness in any given situation. Moreover, without some kind of a balance in these aspects of practical wisdom, the kind of learning that can be generated in a teaching encounter will be limited. For instance, in-depth, subject-matter knowledge alone may lead to a very erudite lecture to a group, but without knowledge of the learning needs of that group, it is possible (or likely) that the level of this talk will be pitched inappropriately. Finally, it is also important to note, that the quest to know more about self, student, and subject will always change, depending on the context or situation in which a teaching and learning encounter occurs. For instance, in any given teaching context, there will be diverse determinants of what occurs: a different physical context, differences in students, and different external mandates pressing in on the action. Thus, the development of practical wisdom in teaching is ongoing; one can never have complete self knowledge, complete knowledge of students, or complete knowledge of subject, in any given situation.

Although we attempt to prepare doctors who begin the MA programme to encounter our focus on practical wisdom as foregrounded over practical 'techniques' of teaching, that approach is usually at odds with their viewpoint and stance at the beginning of the course. This is due to their experiences as clinicians, immersed in a world heavily dominated by the positivistic paradigm of evidence-based medicine. It is a learning journey for all course participants to perceive how a focus on understanding oneself as a teacher, through a deep analysis of different aspects of one's practice, could be functionally useful. The first year of the programme is a particularly crucial phase in this development. The following account of learning illustrates this experience of transition, which is mentioned in more, or less, detail by all participants:

> I have to say, when I embarked on it, I thought it would be very much more practical in terms of 'these are useful techniques for running a small group seminar or putting a lecture together'. When I embarked on it, I didn't really think that it was going to go quite as . . . deep as it did do. And it took me quite a while to settle into that, to see how that might help (Doctor A).

When asked about their experience of the course, in relation to their expectations of it, all nine doctors talked about the difficulties they experienced in coming to grips with the course readings. In particular, they commented on feeling frustrated and overwhelmed at the beginning of the course, as they encountered texts that seemed to be written in an entirely new language. It was not simply the words used by the authors of these educational texts, but the way theories were presented; the manner of presentation seemed unnecessarily long-winded and abstruse, as can be seen in the following comments:

> I had to do it [course reading] with a dictionary because I didn't know what pedagogy was, and I didn't know what a huge number of words were, and it struck me that there were far too many words used. It's a bit like that film of Mozart where he says 'well it's very nice but there are far too many notes' (Doctor D).

> Initially it was a bit of shock, the first article or two, how on earth do people write like this? Because we'd never seen writing like that in our lives before, and reading it was a nightmare because when you've not seen something like that you can't even process it, your brain is not used to it (Doctor E).

It would be possible to take these comments at face value, and see them simply as a critique of the writing style of educational researchers and theorists. Whilst it is true that not all educational research is well written (and, thus, as a course team we need to select supporting literature very carefully), I think that this theme of feeling 'at sea' as a reader of the course texts can also be understood as a commentary on the difficulty of making a transition from the quantitative paradigm, which dominates in the medical field, to the qualitative paradigm, which frames the field of education. To paint a picture of the differences between these fields, using a very broad brush, we can say that the quantitative paradigm is shaped by the realist ontology – a belief that there is an objective reality 'out there', and that the aim of research is to illuminate this 'ultimate truth'. The qualitative paradigm, on the other hand, is founded upon a constructivist ontology – the belief that there is no such thing as an 'ultimate truth', because individuals and groups inevitably construct aspects of this reality through their interpretation of it. I think the difficulties the doctors talk about in relation to the course readings are a window on to a tension they feel as they encounter the educational field of research, characterised by its own peculiar discourse, fuzzy boundaries, and a privileging of learning from single outlier cases, rather than the general or average case privileged in the quantitative paradigm. Central to this journey into educational research is one of becoming used to a more discursive style of analysis than that which is favoured within the quantitative world. Whereas research in the quantitative sphere goes (or at least purports to go!) in a straight line from hypothesis to data-gathering, analysis, and implications for practice, a research study in the qualitative sphere can be more circular and iterative, cycling between a research question, data (which may be empirical or conceptual), and analysis (Denzin and Lincoln 2005). As one doctor put it:

> I just thought it [the course reading] was unnecessarily long-winded, but you kind of acclimatise to that. And I think once you get into the way of thinking and language, it's a little bit like the tippy toe I had dipped into philosophy in various ways: *it's just a different way of thinking* (Doctor D, my emphasis).

Thus, the reaction to the course texts as being 'difficult to read' can be understood as part of the process of a shifting stance, away from seeing teaching development as straightforward 'technique development', towards a perspective, in which learning to teach is felt to be a much more multi-faceted and multi-directional process. The educational theories to which doctors are introduced through the course readings pose difficulties, because these theories inevitably challenge doctors' views of what constitutes good or effective teaching, and thereby raise all kinds of new questions about education in clinical settings. As I outline in the next section, the practice of conducting research into teaching is one that the course team presents as starting with reflection on oneself as teacher and learner. Particularly important to this process of self-study is reflection on the moral substratum that shapes practice – the idiosyncratic set of beliefs, values, and ideals that each of us holds as teachers (and, indeed, simply as human beings), both consciously and unconsciously, and which exerts a very powerful effect on our practice (Barnes 1993; Pajares 1992; Penlington 2006; Richardson 1994).

## Destination, Teacher Change?
## First Stop: Beliefs and Values

It is important to note that the group of doctors who complete the MA Education in Clinical Settings are self-selected, in that they apply to participate in the course because they want to improve their teaching practice. Some start the course because of a feeling that they have reached a plateau or transition point in their careers, and view the development of their teaching practice as a form of career rejuvenation:

> It can be quite boring if you're just a clinician for 30 years or whatever it is, it's such a repetitive thing, so you need something else to make you

get up in the morning and want to go to work, other than seeing just an outpatient clinic, and it's nice to think that you've got a dual role, or more importantly, that you are recognised by people as having a certain skill (Doctor F).

Other doctors are drawn to the MA course because they see it as a means of answering questions or concerns that they have long had about their teaching practice, but which they have not been able to work through in the course of their day-to-day practice:

I came in with a view that it would challenge some of my dogmas, uncomfortable as that might be. But I think I was open to thinking, 'well actually, if I look at my dogmas, they've got me so far but they're not getting me any further' (Doctor G).

MA students viewed development of their teaching, therefore, as a valuable part of their continuing professional development. What we see in the excerpts above is that doctors entered the course, feeling that they had gone as far as they could in developing their practice independently, and so they were looking for a new experience to provide a greater understanding of teaching and learning in clinical settings. As outlined in the previous section, the way in which the MA works to facilitate this change and development – through focusing on the practical wisdom of teaching – is a method which ran counter to many course participants' initial expectations as to what would constitute development in teaching.

Central to this process of change is that of 'excavating' teaching practice, to reveal the complex, and often conflicting, sets of beliefs and ideals that underpin and shape it. This excavation of practice is necessary, because it is through exploring the moral substratum to teaching practice that teachers, in whatever field they are working, can begin to understand the sources for the inevitable inconsistencies between what Argryis and Schön (1975) have termed 'espoused values', and 'values in use'. This is not because teachers are lazy, or chronic self-deceivers; it is simply that teaching practice is often influenced by a set of priorities of which we are not consciously aware (Barnes 1993, 15). Operating beneath the level of our conscious awareness, the moral substratum to our practice is a powerful determinant of what we do as a teacher, as well as being a potential block to change or development in that practice (Penlington 2006). Indeed, the less aware we are of the values, beliefs, and ideals, upon which our practice is founded, the less able we are to make changes to that practice. For example, a doctor may hold the ideal that it is best practice to involve all clinicians actively in dialogue about cases during a ward-round; however, through inquiring into her practice she may find that she regularly quashes or curtails the contributions made by the nurse member of the team. There may be any number of reasons for this dissonance. For instance, it may be that careful analysis of this pattern by the doctor reveals that, although she holds the ideal of involving all members of the team, a more deeply held belief, namely that doctors need to be seen to be knowledgeable and 'in charge', often works in opposition to it.

Interestingly, most of the doctors' comments about the effect of the programme were along the lines that it had not overtly *changed* their beliefs and ideals about teaching but, instead, had made them much more aware, both of the presence of this moral substratum, and of the different ways that it shaped their practice as educators:

> I'm not sure it's changed them [my beliefs and values] but it's made them more conscious, and quite a lot of the early modules were about exploring our values, considering how they applied to the medical education role that we had, and what I became very aware of is that my values and beliefs as a person underpin what I do as a doctor and as an educator actually (Doctor D).

> The course made us question our assumptions, things that you had never really thought about. And then you start to question all sorts of other things that you make assumptions about. And that is good, and it certainly helps, so, you definitely go on a journey (Doctor H).

Some researchers question the emphasis placed on teacher reflection within the field of education, arguing that it is akin to narcissistic navel-gazing, rather than a process likely to result in quantifiable developments in the way a teacher fosters student learning. My experience as a teacher, learner, and educational researcher runs counter to this point of view; it shows that the kind of reflection outlined in this section – what I term deep reflection on practice (a form that inevitably occurs post-hoc, when one has a moment to consider what has transpired and, often, to talk to a colleague) – is vital to the process of teacher learning. It is through this study of practice that teachers become aware of how their patterns and habits of practice affect the learners with whom they work. In other words, teacher reflection of the kind I am setting out is not narcissistic, because the only way of judging whether one has 'done well' as a teacher, is to consider the effect of teaching on students. This theme is further developed in the following section.

## Self-reflection: a Shift in Stance

The results of the present study indicate that a process of reflective inquiry into their own practice helped the doctors move from a focus on 'self as teacher' towards a stance whereby the student occupied more of the centre stage. This is what we see in the following excerpts (illustrative of a general trend across all those interviewed): that the doctors felt that, through completing the course, they had undergone a change in stance from a focus on *teaching*, towards a focus on *learning*.

> I think quite a good insight from the course, which before the course I had never ever thought of, that the learner had a perspective . . . I mean I never consciously thought about it. Maybe I thought 'yes, he or she has come to learn something', so the fact that they have some needs and you have to try to attend to them, like following their agenda rather than following yours, that concern never occurred to me (Doctor E).

> It took me a while to bring out what I feel is really important is the relationship between the teacher and learner, and how they approach learning together, and how important the dynamics are between them: it can't either be the teacher or the learner, it has to be that two-way transfer of information (Doctor A).

Another way of describing this shift in perspective, or stance, is to see it as a movement beyond teaching as performance towards one in which the teacher's focus is on understanding and meeting the needs of the learner. The 'teacher as performance' mode is much more a concern about your own action as a teacher, and how others perceive you. By contrast, focusing on teaching as meeting learners' needs is a perspective in which the teachers are interested, not so much in their performance, but with practising in a way that maximises the learning potential for students. Teaching in this way, therefore, is less about performance and much more to do with enabling students.

In summary, what we see is that the type of reflection on practice that occurs within the MA programme makes teachers inquire into their teaching, not as an end in itself, but as a means to an end: that of facilitating student learning. This shift may sound simple, but as the doctors interviewed for this project noted, it is characterised not so much by becoming more certain about the correct teaching method or technique to use in any given situation, but rather by a process of getting into the habit of continually asking questions about one's practice:

> If I was to pick one thing that the MA taught me (plus, you know, QESP) . . . it is about being reflective, to always be slightly dissatisfied with what you're doing and question how can I make it better? I think that's the important thing (Doctor F).

> It definitely makes you more thoughtful, more questioning. You actually think about how things could be different; what you might do differently and try to appraise the education that you actually are doing (Doctor H).

> I think I spend more time thinking about what happened, which is something I think all of us do every day, but it's become much more focused on trying to see how things could have been better, or what might have been different (Doctor I).

Informing doctors interested in applying for a place on the MA course that, at the end of this course, they will most likely be asking more questions about teaching than they asked at the beginning, is unlikely to be successful as a marketing strategy. However, this effect of the programme is central to its success, because it is one in which participants become researchers of their own practice – a process which, once commenced, becomes an ongoing journey of development, rather than something that ends at the conclusion of the programme. Moreover, as detailed in the next section, the doctors interviewed for this study all noted that the process of becoming researchers of their teaching practice also had a significant impact on how they approached their clinical work.

## The Impact of the MA: Teaching and Beyond

When describing the effect of the MA programme on their practice, the nine doctors interviewed for this study talked about its influence as one that affected not only their teaching practice, but also their clinical practice. This is not surprising, since the educational and the clinical roles of a doctor are very much interlinked (Pugsley and McCrorie 2007), as highlighted in the following excerpt:

> It's such an integral part of doing medicine is to teach, and I think it hasn't always historically been done well, the teaching bit of it . . . but it is so integral to being a doctor is being able to explain, being able to communicate, and whether that's with your patient or whether that's with a trainee, it's just very similar (Doctor G).

The effect of conducting research on their teaching practice, therefore, also involved some kind of study of, and change in, the doctors' clinical practice. For most, this change was about becoming more aware of the educational dimensions of their roles in clinical settings, such as clinics and ward-rounds, as well as within multi-professional team settings. Alongside this awareness was a growing desire to endeavour to practise in such a way so as to maximise the learning that could occur in these situations:

> I think it has affected every part of my practice. For example with the patients, people who come in, I now look at their understanding in a different way, and I think I use some of the principles I learned here in my communication with them . . . So I think that it's affected every part of what I do; in a good way, and I think in a very significant way (Doctor H).

> I think it's about practice being more thoughtful, more considered, looking for opportunities, because they're everywhere, to learn and making that something that people are more conscious of, being more self aware, myself as a doctor and a teacher and encouraging people to be so for themselves (Doctor D).

As noted earlier, one way of describing this change in practical stance through the MA programme is as a paradigm shift on the part of course participants. Whereas previously many of the participants had been steeped in the positivistic paradigm, in which research is conducted via quantitative methods such as double-blind, randomised, controlled trials, the MA Education in Clinical Settings immerses participants in the constructivist paradigm, where it is recognised that there is no 'pure truth', because knowledge is always constructed by agents. This paradigm presents the doctors with a different way of researching practice, one in which the subjective aspect of knowledge is recognised, not as a flaw, but as something to be studied and questioned. The MA is thus focused less on providing course participants with neat answers about education, and more on developing their ability to ask the right kinds of questions. The following quotes show how some of the doctors experienced this paradigm shift, and the effect it had on their practice as doctor-teachers:

So I think the MA helped me on many, many levels, not just in trying to become a better teacher but in answering lots of questions that I had about my practice, about consultants' practice, about protocol-driven practice, about evidence-based practice, because you can have protocols and evidence but they should be as guidelines rather than following them blindly (Doctor E).

And the other thing that was quite interesting was that my colleague, who's also very interested in education, consultant colleague, commented about halfway through the Masters that, she said 'you're much more open to being questioned' and she said 'you're much more open with your ideas and more willing to share them' (Doctor D).

Medicine has become very atomised, quantitative, positivistic if you like, and you know that for some people that fits very well with their subject or what they do, but the humanities aspect of medicine, I think, is not embraced as much as it should be, certainly in my training and my experience, and actually this course clearly, from the stance it takes, puts that centre stage, I think (Doctor G).

It has also changed the way I would look at science, and it's got me reading more about the philosophy behind science . . . I think that affects me as a person, it takes off that rigidity that a certain type of thinking might bring, and makes you more open to other fields (Doctor H).

As can be seen from the above comments, the effect of the MA programme was not just one of creating more questions in participants' minds. If this is all that the programme had achieved, it would have been a very disorienting and unsatisfactory experience for the doctors who completed it. Alongside generating questions about practice, the programme provided participants with a research framework in which to inquire into these questions. So, rather than existing as a series of worries and anxieties about difficulties or problems with teaching, course participants could develop their questions into structured studies of educational practice. Evaluating the impact on educational practice of the research conducted by course alumni in their local setting lies beyond the remit of this chapter. Yet, the interviews with the doctors clearly show that they left the course feeling that they were capable of leading educational change in their local setting in the future. This is interesting, because our ongoing dialogues with the students and alumni of the MA show that, although doctors seldom begin the programme with the aim of wanting to research and change educational practice, by the end of the three-year course, most are very keen to take on some kind of informal or formal leadership role, and to continue to conduct educational research. The following excerpts are typical of how the doctors talked about the long-term effect of the MA:

I think it has helped me develop within medical education within the trust, and that I can see that there are more opportunities further down that route as well, so there are other medical education lead posts for example which potentially I would consider now that I have not only the experience, but also the qualifications to go for, which perhaps previously I might have felt 'well I know quite a lot about that but I don't have any evidence of that' (Doctor F).

The MA has also helped me to think more in terms of trying to evaluate what's happening, so in a very broad way I think it's made me want to do a little bit of research on what's happening, not just see it happen but also evaluate it, investigate it a little bit more, so it's made me more focused in terms of wanting to do research (Doctor I).

I will be getting involved in further qualitative research to develop my practice, and continuing to inquire into how I can become a more effective educator. This course will also greatly improve my work as a Partner in PMETB in certification panels, evaluating deaneries and programmes etc (Doctor C).

What we see from these responses is evidence that the MA course worked, not simply as a means of making the participants more reflective about their own practice as teachers, but also as a way of expanding their practical wisdom in teaching. In other words, it has made them more curious about the complex ways in which the teacher, student, and subject come together in specific contexts, as well as making them more knowledgeable about how to engage in structured inquiry of this complex relationship, so as to develop education in their local situation.

## Conclusion

Although a relative newcomer to the field of PGME, I am no neophyte in the field of education. And my experience in both fields, combined with conversations with doctors in our programmes in KSS, is the grounds for my recognition that we are at a crossroads in PGME. We undoubtedly have a better understanding that postgraduate doctors need clearly defined educational pathways, in order to ensure their effectiveness and safety as clinicians. Yet, the understanding that the doctors who teach this next generation also need to be able to access high-quality programmes to develop their teaching practice, seems to be less accepted in the field of PGME.

Whilst there is clearly a place for teaching workshops aimed at updating doctors on the 'latest and greatest' teaching techniques, these interventions are unlikely to catalyse deep and sustained changes to educational practice in PGME. This small-scale study provides evidence that clinical education, Masters level programmes, which are carefully structured to engage doctors in a deep inquiry of their teaching, do have significant positive effects on their practice, as well as giving doctors an opportunity to form an identity as leaders and change agents within their local education setting. This evidence points to a significant corollary. Given the importance of an increased educational leadership capacity to the continued improvement of teaching and learning within the PGME field, there is need for wider recognition of the role that postgraduate courses, such as this MA Education in Clinical Settings, can play in this developmental process.

# References

Argryis, C., and D. A. Schön. 1975. *Theory in Practice: Increasing Professional Effectiveness*. San Francisco: Jossey-Bass Publishers.

Avalos, B. In press. Teacher Professional Development in Teaching and Teacher Education over Ten Years. *Teaching and Teacher Education*.

Barnes, D. 1993. The Significance of Teachers' Frames for Teaching. In *Teachers and Teaching: from Classroom to Reflection*, eds. T. Russell and H. Munby, 9-32. London: Falmer Press.

Borko, H. 2004. Professional Development and Teacher Learning: *Mapping the Terrain. Educational Researcher* 33 (8): 3-15.

Denzin, N. K., and Y. S. Lincoln. 2005. The Discipline and Practice of Qualitative Research. In *The Sage Handbook of Qualitative Research*, eds. N. K. Denzin and Y. S. Lincoln, 1-32. Thousand Oaks, California: Sage.

Kogana, J. R., and J. A. Shea. 2007. Course Evaluation in Medical Education. *Teaching and Teacher Education* 23 (3): 251–264.

Lieberman, A. 1994. Teacher Development: Commitment and Challenge. In *Teacher Development and the Struggle for Authenticity: Professional Growth and Restructuring in the Context of Change*, eds. P. P. Grimmett and J. Neufeld, 15-30. New York: Teachers College Press.

Pajares, M. F. 1992. Teacher Beliefs and Educational Research: Cleaning Up a Messy Construct. *Review of Educational Research* 62 (3): 307-332.

Penlington, C. 2006. Teachers Reasoning Practically: a Philosophical Analysis of How Teachers Develop their Practice through Dialogue with Others. Doctoral dissertation, Education, University of Michigan, Ann Arbor.

Pugsley, L., and P. McCrorie. 2007. Improving Medical Education: Improving Patient Care. *Teaching and Teacher Education* 23: 314-322.

Richardson, V. 1994. The Consideration of Teacher Beliefs. *In Teacher Change and the Staff Development Process*, ed. V. Richardson, 90-108. New York: Teachers College Press.

Richardson, V. 2003. The Dilemmas of Professional Development. *Phi Delta Kappan* 84 (5): 401-406.

Sockett, H. 1993. *The Moral Base for Teacher Professionalism*. New York: Teachers College Press.

Stein, M. K., M. S. Smith, and E. A. Silver. 1999. The Development of Professional Developers: Learning to Assist Teachers in New Settings in New Ways. *Harvard Educational Review* 69 (3): 237-269.

# Techniques and Technologies: Developing Curriculum-Led Simulation

In recent years Kent, Surrey and Sussex Postgraduate Medical Deanery [KSS] has developed new provision for simulation in postgraduate medical education [PGME]. Here, I consider the historical development of simulation in a range of medical contexts and the evolution of KSS's approach to its provision as part of our educational practices. The KSS approach to simulation is consistent with the principles and values described in Chapter 2 and is informed by theoretical perspectives on simulation, such as notions of realism and fidelity within teaching and learning contexts. By taking a 'biopsy' of KSS's current provision of simulation I offer an overview of the initiatives and strategies used to ensure the active involvement of clinicians across our Local Education Providers [LEPs] and thus, to achieve local creativity, diversity, and ownership within an overall KSS Operational Strategy. Finally, I consider how curriculum-led simulation [CLS] might more effectively enhance standards in PGME and identify emergent practice. My overall proposal is that simulation should prioritise the collaborative learning of all participants within a context that puts patient safety first.

KSS Education Department began to oversee and quality-manage simulation on behalf of South East Coast Strategic Health Authority [SEC] in Autumn 2006. The requirement was to ensure a unified approach to the various technology-driven initiatives emerging in medical education within the region. This work required interacting with a wide range of partners and stakeholders within LEPs. It also required representing KSS nationally, as part of the Department of Health's [DH] Study on Simulation Provision in 2009, and internationally, by attending Society for Simulation in Healthcare events. When I joined the Education Department in September 2008, I became KSS Lead for Simulation, responsible for the strategic growth of simulation provision and for unifying the community of simulation practice across our region. My previous role within a small college of the University of London had allowed me to develop some understandings of the relationships between technologies and learning which I thought might be transferable to PGME. However, I was also aware of the need to be flexible in developing an approach to project management that would meet the particular challenges of PGME.

KSS has an established relationship with London Deanery and its Simulation and Technology-enhanced Learning Initiative [STeLI] project. In 2008 London Deanery invested substantial capital and recurrent funding for equipment and staff in STeLI as one of its flagship initiatives. The simulation provision made by KSS, and described below, is rather different to STeLI. However, the KSS approach may be of more practical use in regions where postgraduate doctors are spread across wide geographical areas and provision is being developed within tight financial constraints.

Both KSS and London Deanery support South Thames Foundation School [STFS] postgraduate doctors, who rotate through hospitals across London and SEC. Provision of simulation for postgraduate doctors within STFS is a key focus of our work. In Autumn 2006 KSS began to develop its CLS approach, initially as a pilot for 120 Foundation Year One [F1] postgraduate doctors. We developed a relationship with three specialist, high-tech simulation centres at St. George's, Barts and the London School of Medicine and Dentistry, and Brighton and Sussex Medical School. Attendance at KSS simulation events at these three centres grew from 120 F1 postgraduate doctors in 2007, to 300 in 2009, and then to 491 in 2010. This attendance has levelled out at 496 F1 postgraduate doctors in 2011.

F1 postgraduate doctors are not registered with the General Medical Council [GMC], and so it is not ethical or legal for them to work independently with patients. Simulation is the only means of allowing them to practise stabilising the condition of a very ill patient. This is what we mean by CLS: an approach which uses simulation specifically to teach elements of the curriculum which cannot be taught in real-life clinical practice. KSS worked with our three specialist providers to develop a one-day simulation event, in which F1 postgraduate doctors explored the experience of trying to stabilise a very ill 'patient', while seeking telephone advice from a Specialist Registrar [SpR], and assisting in diagnosing the patient's condition. The high-tech dummies used in these events, their skilled operators, and experienced role-players make the simulation very realistic. From 2008 STFS required all F1 postgraduate doctors to undertake CLS in order to be signed-off.

Concurrently, KSS began to develop provision of CLS within LEPs. By 2010, seven out of eleven LEPs had developed F1 CLS. The remaining four LEPs have received pump-priming funding from KSS to develop similar provision by the end of 2011. Until then, CLS for their F1 postgraduate doctors is being provided in partnership with Brighton and Sussex University Hospital and with the Royal Surrey County Hospital. KSS Education Department believes that local provision of simulation, firmly embedded in LEPs, is more cost-effective than the use of high-tech centres alone. As the National Health Service [NHS] faces increasing financial pressures, and as pressures on service delivery increase, it is becoming difficult and expensive to release groups of postgraduate doctors for large blocks of time, to travel to distant sites. As long as local provision is carefully quality-managed, it offers good access, a means of developing diverse and creative approaches, as well as affordability and continuity.

⊙⊙

# Theoretical Perspectives on Simulation

Simulation has been used extensively for teaching and learning in areas where practice poses danger to human life, or where there is a clear cost benefit in developing skills prior to their application. This is particularly true in military contexts, and in technology-rich contexts, such as aviation, marine exploration, and outer-space exploration, where sophisticated and expensive machinery is used. Healthcare practitioners have taken up some of the ideas and approaches developed in these contexts, but in PGME the aspects of practice that lie beyond the development of technical skills are particularly important. In KSS, we have sought ways to ensure that, wherever possible, simulation offers our doctors a chance to develop their wider professional understandings – gnosis, as well as skills – episteme (see Chapter 2).

Medicine has a long history of practising on models of the human form, which is simulation at its most fundamental. Many historical artefacts, from phrenology busts to pigskin-suturing models, bear witness to this, and reveal philosophical attitudes to 'knowing' about biological aspects of the human condition. Building on this inheritance, the twentieth century has seen a rapid growth in technological developments within simulation practice. This has reflected the way in which microchip technology has revolutionised clinical procedures, especially in the 'front-line' specialties of Emergency Care, Surgery, and Anaesthetics. Increasingly, medical simulators are being developed and deployed to teach therapeutic and diagnostic procedures, as well as medical concepts and clinical decision making. Simulators have been developed for training procedures ranging from basic procedures, such as drawing blood, to laparoscopic surgery and surgical rehearsal. Simulators are also used to research and develop new tools for therapies, treatments, and early diagnosis across all medical specialties.

Ideally, medicine is learned in practice. However, simulation is indispensable as a means of providing postgraduate doctors with experience to which they do not have access in practice. This is the case in the KSS CLS provision for F1 postgraduate doctors, where simulation allows them to practise independently managing very sick patients, stabilising their condition and contributing to diagnosis. It applies equally to learning opportunities that might be considered to be above the level of qualification of individual postgraduate doctors, especially in acute clinical contexts. Further, since a significant part of effective medical practice is about routine matters, such as timely monitoring and replacement of fluids, and effective communication between team members, simulation scenarios can also play a very important role in 'getting the basics right'.

There is a broad spectrum of approaches to teaching and learning through simulation. In many contexts, simulation is an educational process derived from a 'technical-rational' approach to understanding (de Cossart and Fish 2005). Nevertheless, in KSS, we have worked on the assumption that simulation might usefully be adapted to meet the needs of a profession in which the arts, the humanities, the sciences, and new technologies meet and are of equal importance. Simulation should be understood as a broad and flexible teaching method, that might embrace many dimensions of contemporary healthcare education. It can provide postgraduate doctors with structured opportunities to learn about essential aspects of clinical practice, such as doctor-patient and doctor-doctor communication, managing teams, and other human factors that impact on patient safety. If we accept that 'knowledge is constructed and made meaningful by the context in which it is acquired' (Farmer et al 1992, 46), we will need to bear in mind that there are differences between the reality of performance in practice, and the reality of simulation. However, this difference in realities is helpful, since it represents the intentional use of the imagination by individuals to assist themselves in dealing with complex, difficult, new, or different circumstances. In this sense, simulation might be compared with reflective practice, which also aims to prepare the learner for real-life situations in the future. Thus, simulation might be extended appropriately to realms such as assessment, re-accreditation, and the support of postgraduate doctors with additional learning needs.

As Pearson (2009, 11) has identified, 'patient safety has become a key focus for clinical service in the UK NHS, and now has both organisational structures and a research agenda to consolidate what it means in practice. There is not yet a strong evidence base for the ways in which "patient safety" is understood and applied during training'. Simulation might be helpful in bringing together self-directed study with learning in clinical settings, and thereby contributing to the patient safety agenda. This might be particularly effective in a context where the European Working Time Regulations [EWTR] make it challenging to balance educational needs with service needs.

For learning to be at its most effective, learners need to enter into a type of emotional and intellectual contract with the experience so that they can embrace its value as 'real'. In his *Biographia Literaria*, Coleridge called this 'the willing suspension of disbelief'. His concern was that the world of the imagination had fallen out of intellectual fashion in the eighteenth century, as the educated classes embraced science and a rationalist perspective on human understanding:

> My endeavours should be directed to persons and characters supernatural, or at least romantic, yet so as to transfer from our inward nature a human interest and a semblance of truth sufficient to procure for these shadows of imagination that willing suspension of disbelief for the moment, which constitutes poetic faith (*Biographia Literaria*, 160).

The concept of 'the willing suspension of disbelief' operates powerfully in art forms with performance and representational dimensions, such as theatre and cinema. Thus, we can understand the extension of this idea to the realm of simulation, as learners are immersed in scenarios as participants or as observers, and actively create their interior meanings of these scenarios. They may later share these with colleagues, and thus co-construct new meanings.

Research and development related to medical simulation often concerns itself with making faithful reproductions of the real, in a bid to authenticate and validate experience in its specialist-centre contexts. Multi-million-pound investment in specialist centres is framed around the assumption that high-fidelity simulation experiences are the only way to 'keep it real' and make simulation relevant to learners. I would argue that providing effective learning opportunities in response to the curriculum needs of postgraduate doctors, is more important than technological wizardry. In this sense, 'relevance to practice in real-life contexts' has to be the measure. Often, postgraduate doctors need first and foremost to develop confidence in straightforward life-preserving measures, such as the administration and management of fluids. The use of simulation to develop postgraduate doctors' confidence in such everyday areas of practice is just as valuable as its use in relation to more unusual and technologically advanced scenarios. Approaching simulation as one dimension of a constructivist process, where learners actively contribute to making meanings, is important if we are to develop training that is 'done with' rather than 'done to'. As Marks-Maran puts it: 'It is not the simulation that makes the learning; it is the pedagogy of simulation that makes the learning' (Marks-Maran n.d.).

Discussions about the efficacy of simulation often focus on issues concerning the level of realism and fidelity. Exponents of simulation commonly assert that only the truthful reproduction of 'the real' can generate a realistic learning environment. They operate from the supposition that, for learning to take place, participants need to 'believe' in the experience and allow themselves to be immersed in an immediate environment, which is a truthful and credible representation of the workplace. Fidelity may be understood as the degree to which the characteristics of the simulation or simulator match the characteristics of a real-life clinical encounter. This suggests that to maximise the representation of the real, both physical and psychological dimensions need to be addressed. However, as Coleridge indicates, 'suspension of disbelief' is achieved primarily through an imaginative engagement, which does not necessarily require a high degree of literalism and may, indeed, be constrained by it. Thus, as contemporary drama demonstrates, the ways in which an experience of 'the real' is brought about may vary from complex, highly naturalistic sets, with extensive use of theatre properties, to rooms empty of anything apart from the people creating and observing the simulation. Effective simulation can take place with a minimum of technical equipment.

'Hands-on' learning opportunities are crucial in helping postgraduate doctors to develop expediency in their practice, particularly in craft specialties such as surgery. One of the traditional means of providing postgraduate doctors with a chance to 'practise with a scalpel and needle' has been 'part-task' trainers. These desktop simulators enable learners to practise skills like cutting and suturing on dedicated apparatus manufactured from pigskin or synthetic materials. While these technologies can serve a useful purpose, perhaps their placement on worktops in skills laboratories removes a degree of fidelity, which means they are of less value to the reality of work in theatre. For example, in his recent work, Roger Kneebone has 'mounted' simulated wounds on actors' limbs. This ensures that learners have to develop skills of manual dexterity alongside coping mechanisms for dealing with emotionally demanding patients. It also brings into play communication skills and thinking under pressure, to deal with realistic characterisations from role-players acting as stereotypical 'standardised' patients. Here, Kneebone has re-imagined traditional elements of PGME and repositioned them in the context of contemporary medical practice.

⚭

## Quality Management and Leadership

Quality management for simulation is based on the principle that provision should arise from curriculum needs; this is the CLS approach. Since there are National Curriculum Frameworks [NCFs] for the Foundation Programme [Foundation] and for specialties, CLS is based on an explicit set of standards that reflect the intentions and purposes of the GMC and the medical Royal Colleges [Royal Colleges]. Chapters 1 and 3 describe the structures of Local Academic Boards [LABs] and Local Faculty Groups [LFGs], through which KSS manages its Education Contract with LEPs. Simulation is part of these contractual and governance systems, which means that there is a robust management structure and a clear set of quality standards for simulation in KSS. This is particularly important, since the distributed model of provision that we use means that we support the development of a wide range of approaches to simulation. However, the quality-management structure within which they all operate, ensures a consistent learning experience for postgraduate doctors across KSS.

Internally, a Steering Group is the central management and leadership platform for simulation within KSS. It includes a clinical Lead, the responsible Assistant Dean Education [ADE], an Associate Director of the Foundation School, two Consultant-level Simulation Trust Leads and a director of SimMed, an organisation based at the Royal Surrey County Hospital, that leads on simulation. In this way, we seek to be representative of our stakeholder community. The Steering Group produces and revises an Operational Strategy, which consists of three strands of provision, and aims to maximise postgraduate doctors' exposure to KSS CLS. One strand is the use of high-tech simulation centres, described above. The second strand is mobile provision; its approach is arts-informed, flexible and low-tech. A specialist team collaborates with LEPs and visits them to provide a specific, tailored simulation experience, often one that the LEP would find difficult to develop on its own. The third strand comprises local provision that is entirely LEP-owned and facilitated by the LFG. It has the advantage that the LEP's and LFG's medical policies and practices can be reflected in the scenarios they write for their postgraduate doctors.

At local level, LEP Leads for simulation sit on the LAB, and bring specific expertise to bear within the institution. This role attracts 0.25 hours of Planned Activity time in the LEP Lead's Job Plan, which ensures recognition of their work by the LEP. LEP Leads support and develop simulation through the LFGs, and make an important contribution to locally owned provision by bringing together a range of their colleagues from the healthcare professions. In some LEPs, this is organised as a simulation LFG, reporting to the LAB, and attended by representatives from each of the LEP's clinical departments.

Complementing this structure, Specialty Leads for simulation were appointed from 2010 onwards. Appointments have been made in Anaesthetics, Emergency Medicine, Obstetrics and Gynaecology, General Medicine, Paediatrics, Psychiatry, Radiology, and Surgery. Specialty Leads work closely with specialty schools in developing CLS.

Developing a community of practice in simulation was a central tenet of our strategy and policy. Adhering to the principle of shared ownership is crucial in ensuring the investment and 'buy-in' of stakeholders from across the KSS region. In practice, this is manifest in consultation processes and in the collaborative development of the simulation policy. The KSS strategy employs both an LEP-based approach and a Specialty-based approach, which combine to form our community of practice. If we remind ourselves of Wenger's notion of a community of practice as a 'group of people who share a concern, a set of problems, or a passion about a topic, and who deepen their knowledge and expertise in this area by interacting on an ongoing basis' (Wenger et al 2002, 4), then our role is to most effectively facilitate these interactions over time. In the twenty-first century, LEPs and the specialties of the doctors who work within them, are characterised to a greater or lesser extent by an apparent tension between the provision of a free health service to the British public and a sense of competition. The adoption of a market approach to healthcare services by successive governments since the 1970s has created the risk that knowledge might not be shared freely between healthcare organisations. The KSS approach has been to recognise the reality of this competitive arena and to encourage the sharing of practice to drive up standards across the region. We recognise that 'however they accumulate knowledge, they become informally bound by the value that they find in learning together' (Wenger et al 2002, 5).

The process of developing this community of practice began in 2007 with the creation of the KSS Simulation Partnership Group. This comprised a half-day planning conference, where interested parties came together to discuss priorities for our region, with the aim of sharing best practice. This forum proved so successful that a Special Interest Group was established, bringing together the community of practice each year in a series of occasional seminars and consultation events. In 2010, we decided to develop a 'brand identity' for simulation within KSS and established SimNet, our Simulation Network.

Building on this, the KSS Simulation and Faculty Education [SAFE] project targets the wider team of practitioners, whose involvement is crucial if simulation in their LEP is to be effective. The SAFE project was piloted in 2009, and is facilitated by the SimMed team from the Royal Surrey County Hospital. A member of the SAFE team makes an initial needs-assessment visit to ascertain where the full visiting team needs to concentrate its energies in a half-day workshop to be held at a later date. The SAFE Project provides an experienced and realistic overview and pragmatic approach to meeting the challenges of centre-owned provision, while enabling effective, collaborative planning, and the delivery of sustainable simulation provision.

Finally, Simulation Quality and Development [SQuaD] visits utilise the practice of observation and 'professional conversation', described in Chapters 4, 5, and 6. A central tenet of the visits is that they are 'done with' rather than 'done to', a collaborative approach that ensures a strong sense of local ownership of simulation practice, and one that is tailored to recognise local circumstances. The visiting team includes a consultant, an ADE, and a simulation specialist from one of our partner organisations. Feedback from these visits has been highly positive, as colleagues value the opportunity to engage in a professional dialogue with a team that can spread effective practice and celebrate local achievement. A further positive outcome has been the development of a network of simulation practitioners who are able to critique each other's practice in an ongoing dialogue, as part of our community of practice.

## Emergent Practice

The keystone of our emergent practice is a detailed consideration of the most beneficial role that simulation can play in the curriculum, and the way in which teachers and learners can integrate a simulation experience into the rest of their learning: this is our CLS approach. It developed in response to a concern that day visits to high-tech simulation centres might be dislocated from the curriculum, focus more on technology than learning, and utilise 'high-thrill' values rather than reflective ones. So, our practice requires a consultant from the LEP to accompany postgraduate doctors on a day visit to a high-tech simulation centre, so that the experience and knowledge gained from the visit can be linked explicitly to the Local Curriculum in Practice [LCP]. The consultants from the LEPs need to be fully briefed in advance on their role in working alongside the staff in the high-tech centre, if they are to be most effective in meeting the needs of learners. As Alinier (2010,1) recognises, 'it needs to be acknowledged that it is the educators [in this case, simulation facilitators] that are the most important asset in most educational experiences, as simulation technology alone has very limited potential'.

Prior to attending a high-tech simulation centre, postgraduate doctors are required to use pre-course materials to consider how simulation is pertinent to their curriculum and assessment portfolio. The welcome meeting is important in setting the tone of the day, and in setting up the simulation with learners. Learners need to understand that the pedagogical approach requires them to be active learners, and that simulation is best 'done with' rather than 'done to'. Pair and small group work are important educational strategies in this respect; they allow learners to test out ideas and thoughts more intimately than in whole-group discussions. Alinier (2010, 6) asserts that centres need to be proactive in setting up the learning on offer in the simulator as part of the introduction to the experience: 'The educational approach with which simulation tools are used are more important than the tools themselves. To provide a beneficial learning experience, the simulator needs to be used appropriately, that is according to the level of experience of the students, in a friendly and supportive manner'.

Well-written simulation scenarios are the starting point of effective teaching practice. They must be true-to-real-life clinical experience, and provide multiple perspectives if they are to be most effective in providing a robust educational experience. To this end, we write differentiated scenarios collaboratively with the LFG from the learner's LEP. Scenarios provide outlines for postgraduate doctors in the simulator and for those watching; for all participating healthcare professionals in facilitator roles; and for the lead clinician / facilitator of the post-simulation professional conversation.

Since most of our simulation events are provided for numbers of around twelve learners, it is important that learners remain active when they are not in the simulator. Our centres have developed models of 'targeted watching' that enable viewers to take responsibility for particular aspects of the scenario, such as doctor-to-doctor communication, differential diagnoses at various points of the scenario, and team communication practices. Active viewers are more likely to be participative learners, who can then take their newly generated data in to the professional conversation with a sense of authority.

It is the critical feedback of the professional conversation that is considered to 'close the learning loop'. A shared, reflective approach extends the dimensions of the professional conversation, and provides a contrast to traditional notions of 'debrief'. Shared reflection is enhanced when learners have a chance to pause for thought to reflect on the experience. Kuiper's research provides convincing evidence that simulation offers a valuable teaching and learning strategy to promote situated cognition and clinical reasoning, and that it teaches learners to solve problems. 'Structured debriefing activities that develop clinical reasoning following high-fidelity patient simulation show that the approach of the educationist is key in facilitating meaningful reflection' (Kuiper 2008). While supporting the general principles expressed here, I believe there is value in considering the nuances of language: the term 'debrief' originated in highly structured meetings of American air crews, who gathered to assess the effectiveness of bombing missions. Such hierarchically organised structures, focused on desensitising groups and individuals to the horrors and alienation of mass destruction, might not be an ideal model for developing an open exchange of thoughts and feelings between postgraduate doctors about the best care for individual patients.

All KSS postgraduate doctors are required to evaluate their experience. This feedback has traditionally taken the form of written, 'white space' evaluation sheets. Our experience is that tick-lists and 'happy-sheets' close down reflection, rather than opening it up. We are now piloting less formal means for learners to feed back on their experiences. A Foundation Year Two [F2] initiative that is currently being piloted employs a blog, so that learners can feed back through informal social networking. Evaluative data from learners might suggest new insights into their needs, which will be helpful in revising and enhancing simulation scenarios in our review processes.

## Conclusions

I have suggested that simulation techniques and technologies should, first and foremost, be considered in the light of their potential for learning in PGME. Rather than simulation being regarded as an end in itself, CLS posits simulation as one of a range of means for teaching the LCP. The KSS simulation community of practice has identified a range of future areas for development in further developing CLS across the region, especially as part of the Education Department's work in curriculum mapping. This collaborative development will make explicit the curricular benchmarks for simulation, which are at present implicit in Royal Colleges' NCFs.

# References

Alinier, G. 2010. *Simulated Practice in Healthcare: Technology and Educational Approach*. Learning Exchange. Westminster.

Coleridge, S. T. 1975. *Biographia Literaria*. Edited by George Watson. London: Dent.

Farmer Jr, J. A., A. Buckmaster and B. LeGrand. Cognitive Apprenticeship: implications for continuing professional education. *New Directions in Adult and Continuing Education*. 55 (Fall 1992): 41-49.

de Cossart, L. and D. Fish. 2005. *Cultivating a Thinking Surgeon*. Shrewsbury: tfm Publishing Ltd.

Kuiper, R. 2008. *Debriefing with the OPT Model of Clinical Reasoning during High Fidelity Patient Simulation*. Berkeley: Electronic Press.

Marks-Maran, D. n.d. *Using Simulation in Nursing Education: Pedagogy, Research and Curriculum*. www.meti.com/uk_wrapup (accessed 22 January, 2011)

Pearson, P. 2009. *Patient Safety in Health Care Professional Educational Curricula: Examining the Learning Experience*. London: HMSO.

Wenger, E., R. McDermott and W. Snyder. 2002. *Cultivating Communities of Practice*. Boston: Harvard Business School.

# Supporting Patients with Learning Disabilities: Power, Empowerment and Voice

## New Imperatives

In response to government initiatives and legislative changes since 2009, postgraduate medical education [PGME] has had to reconsider the way in which its curriculum prepares postgraduate doctors to work with patients with learning disabilities [PLDs]. I should like briefly to rehearse the background to this curriculum change, and then to describe the response made by the Education Department at Kent, Surrey and Sussex Postgraduate Medical Deanery [KSS], simultaneously locating our response within broader contexts of healthcare needs for PLDs.

In 2007, the Mencap report, *Death by Indifference*, catalogued six cases where PLDs had died in UK hospitals. The report stated unequivocally that these patients had not received the quality of care to which they were entitled, simply because they had learning disabilities. In effect, their deaths had been brought about by the indifference of the National Health Service [NHS] towards them. An independent inquiry was launched, and a report from the Ombudsman, entitled *Six Lives: the Provision of Public Services to People with Learning Disabilities* (2009), upheld the Mencap report in three of the six instances. As a direct response to this, in 2009 the government launched the *Valuing People* programme, which aimed to raise awareness of the rights of PLDs in terms of equitable patient care.

Concurrently, a new piece of legislation, the *Corporate Manslaughter and Corporate Homicide Act*, set out a new offence, whereby an organisation may be convicted if 'the way in which its activities are managed or organised causes a death, and amounts to a gross breach of a duty of care to the deceased' (2007, 1). Organisations that fail to comply with the new Act face prosecution, unlimited fines, and the prosecution of senior managers and their staff for gross negligence manslaughter, and culpable homicide. This new legislation implies that, within the NHS, both employers and employees are liable to criminal prosecution in cases where indifference to patients' learning disabilities brings about their death. Literally, the Chief Executive Officers [CEOs] of NHS Trusts, and their doctors and other healthcare workers, may be taken into custody, prosecuted at the expense of the Crown, and serve prison sentences, if found guilty. This is quite different from a system in which patients and their families might take out civil proceedings, at their own expense, if they feel that an NHS organisation has provided inadequate healthcare. Now, the starting point for dealing with such complaints may be the patient and their family reporting neglect to the police, with legal action being carried out by the Crown Prosecution Service, funded by the public purse. The patient's own civil proceedings, to gain monetary compensation, would then follow a successful criminal prosecution, and might be subsumed by it. Although case law in this area remains to be established, experts in the field believe that it represents a high level of potential risk for NHS organisations, their CEOs, and their employees, particularly in the light of the Ombudsman's response to Mencap's report (Sara Chadd, personal communication, July 2010). This new legislation applies to the treatment of all patients, of course, but it is particularly apposite for PLDs, where the ethical duty of care is now very strongly underlined by an increased level of corporate risk.

The KSS response to these new imperatives was to begin by considering the need for curriculum development for the Foundation Programme [Foundation]. We wished to develop a programme, that would enable postgraduate doctors to support PLDs better, and that would promote the rights of PLDs when they interact with healthcare professionals. We recognised the need to be explicit about the current legal position for PLDs, as well as the challenges facing patients, in terms of their lives, their sense of being *different*, and their specific healthcare issues. As a first step, we developed, and offered, a half-day workshop to Foundation doctors in all KSS Local Education Providers [LEPs].

In developing the workshop, I drew on my many years of positive experience in working with children and adults with learning disabilities, both in the UK and in Norway, and in my experience of educating teachers to teach learners with a range of abilities and disabilities. Concurrently with developing and teaching the workshop, I have also been caring for my elderly parent, who has aphasia following a stroke. Aphasia does not damage intelligence, but it does affect how someone can use language, in terms of speaking, understanding what is said, reading, and writing, and in these ways it mimics some of the characteristics of learning disability (National Aphasia Association 2011). Consequently, I have had frequent opportunities to experience the problematics of interactions between medical professionals, and a person who appears to have a learning disability.

# Equality Matters

The legal position in the UK is straightforward, with the rights of individuals to equality being enshrined within legislation, enacted over a period of time, and now encapsulated in the *Equality Act* (2010). However, there is evidence that healthcare provision has some way to go before PLDs are routinely, and regularly, offered equal levels of service in NHS settings. The Michael Report, *Healthcare for All* (DH 2008, 2), highlights grave inequalities:

The evidence shows that there is a significant gap between policy, the law and the delivery of effective health services for people with learning disabilities. There is guidance on the delivery of effective general healthcare for people with learning disabilities, but it is poorly understood, health care services are poorly co-ordinated in relation to the needs of people with learning disabilities and *few providers are taking the essential steps needed to improve practice* [my emphasis].

The most recent statistics indicate that there are almost a million people in England, that is, approximately 2% of the population, who have a diagnosis of learning disability (Emerson and Hatton 2004). Improving patient care for such a large group of people should not be tokenistic, piecemeal, or subject to the so-called 'postcode lottery' of regional fluctuation but should be aligned with national strategies for improving care for all patients.

## Wider Contexts: Stigma and Concealment

There is a growing body of evidence that indicates that those with learning disabilities continue to be stigmatised within the wider community. McArdle (2001) indicates that people with speech, language, and communication difficulties have a broad range of concealed impairments, and he discusses how these impact significantly on their lives. It is common for individuals to begin to withdraw from situations where communication is necessary. They may find this to be emotionally easier than occupying an outsider position, arising from their inability to understand what is going on, their fear of committing a social gaffe, and their consequent feelings of being vulnerable to humiliation. The stigmatisation of individuals, including those with learning disabilities, is regarded as commonplace, as the Royal College of Psychiatrists pointed out in its *Fair Deal for Mental Health Campaign* (2010, 33):

> Discrimination remains endemic throughout the UK, despite many campaigns to eradicate it. For some groups that discrimination is compounded because of the person's race, disability, cultural background or sexuality.

The campaign continued by calling on the NHS to:

> take the lead in reducing discrimination against people with mental health problems and learning disabilities and to ensure that their disability equality schemes adequately address duties in relation to people with mental health problems and learning disabilities.

## Authentic Voices Articulate the Fact of Being Different

### *Relationships*

The preliminary research for the KSS PLD project revealed a paucity of teaching material that included PLDs discussing their interactions with healthcare professionals. We decided, therefore, to capture on film a number of conversations with people who were willing to provide authentic accounts of their experiences. Deciding what to include, and identifying those who would be prepared to assist, was challenging. A series of conversations was finally developed comprising: a young woman with Broca's aphasia (A); a man with Asperger's syndrome and learning disabilities (B); and a woman with cerebral palsy and learning disabilities (C). To ensure that the family and carers' perspectives are included, we also interviewed (C)'s husband, mother and sister.

These short conversations provide exemplars of communication, and the views of individuals, with a range of learning disabilities and conditions. Common themes, such as the desire not to be patronised by healthcare professionals, and individual issues, are identified and discussed in the workshop mentioned at the beginning of this chapter. It is clear that PLDs may face unknown and unfamiliar situations with considerable anxiety, and may exhibit unusual or challenging behaviour. In these circumstances it is crucial for healthcare professionals to create calm and order, so that individuals' anxiety levels can be lowered, as a precondition for providing effective medical treatment. The film clips also highlight that, while those interviewed are aware that there are limitations on their ability to communicate and learn, they are also aware that they are not treated equally.

Two of the film clips demonstrate that family or carers who have frequent, close relationships with PLDs, constantly make adjustments that enable greater interaction. This can reduce their perception of the degree of learning disability experienced by the individual, its impact on them, and its impact on others. We highlight this feature in the workshop, because it can affect the nature and quality of three-way discussions between carers, PLDs, and the doctor attending them. Leading on from this, we consider the need to look beneath surface interactions to develop fuller, more complex understandings. This is particularly important in the contexts of relationships with family and friends. The people in our film clips receive significant support from family members, although (B) is living in the community in supported living accommodation. This input from, and reliance on, family is typical for PLDs, with statistics for England (Emerson and Hatton 2004) identifying that 60% of adults with learning disabilities live with their families. Those statistics also reveal that one in three people with learning disabilities says that they do not have any friends. There may be many individual reasons for this, but there is evidence that fear of feeling like an outsider, which is discussed by (A) in the film clip, is a common reason for diminished social interaction, and a sense of loneliness and otherness.

Interestingly, this feeling of being an outsider or, as she put it, an *alien* is one referred to by Clare Sainsbury, who, as a young woman with Asperger's syndrome, wrote the book *Martian in the Playground* (Sainsbury 2000), where she describes eloquently how alien she, and twenty-five other people with Asperger's syndrome, always felt at school. Luke

Jackson echoes her sentiments in his *Freaks, Geeks and Asperger Syndrome* (2002). This feeling of being an outsider, or different, is a common refrain when talking to people with a learning disability. Perhaps this is a way into a discussion about difference in a way we can all understand? Do doctors feel that PLDs are *other* or outsiders to the healthcare system? Is it possible that doctors also feel like outsiders, when they need to interact with PLDs and their carers?

## Experiencing Pain

Individual sensitivity to pain can vary greatly in PLDs, who may feel either an acute sensitivity and low tolerance to pain, or, conversely, little or no neurological response to pain. Such variations can operate across the full range of sensations, so that people with autistic spectrum disorders, for example, may be acutely sensitive to light, to noise, to taste, to texture, to temperature, or to a combination of these. Further, people with autistic spectrum disorders may feel pain on a continuum; some have a lack of sensitivity, so pain is scarcely felt (even after quite severe injury such as broken bones), while others feel pain acutely (Cooper 1988; Davis and Schunick 2002; Kerr 2007). In our film clips, (B) describes his extremely low pain threshold and, although he is aware that he may be exaggerating the pain due to his anxiety, his response to it is acute. Detecting pain in people with profound learning disabilities is even more complex, as the individuals may be unable to communicate that they are in pain (Astor 2001). Instead, the individual may present as being challenging, or self-injurious, with the resultant risk of diagnostic overshadowing.

## Diagnostic Overshadowing

Diagnostic overshadowing is another, under-discussed, risk faced by PLDs. The term refers to the risk of someone's somatic symptoms being explained away as part of their learning disability. Holland (2000) suggests that assumptions made by doctors regarding behaviour in PLDs, can be a hindrance, both to accurate diagnosis, and to access to equitable and appropriate healthcare. In extreme cases, this may result in life-threatening illnesses being misdiagnosed, or overlooked. Diagnostic overshadowing is also linked with under-diagnosis of mental health problems in PLDs (Jopp and Keys 2001; Mason and Scior 2004). It was considered to be the root cause of lack of treatment in one of the cases in *Death by Indifference* (Mencap 2007, 20), and is highlighted in the Disability Rights Commission's investigation into unequal treatment of people with learning disabilities:

> All the families in the case studies said that they were not listened to by the medical staff treating their sons and daughters. This was the case with Mark's family, who felt that they were consistently ignored when they expressed their concerns. Warren's mother and father asked doctors repeatedly if Warren might have appendicitis or a blocked bowel. But they too felt that their concerns were ignored . . . Warren died within two hours of admission to the hospital. His death certificate lists two causes of his death as: peritonitis following perforation of his appendix, and a paralytic ileus (a bowel blockage caused by a paralysed bowel). These were precisely the conditions about which his parents had repeatedly voiced their suspicions.

This particular case also highlights how the voice of the carer needs to be heard, and their observations of behavioural changes noted, when a PLD cannot articulate their pain. This area of concern is echoed in the case of Hugh, a non-verbal man in his forties, who suffered intense pain for five months for a severe back complaint, as carers and doctors assumed his increasingly challenging behaviour was a result of his learning disability, rather than of a physical medical cause (Flynn 2004). Only his sister's insistence led to an accurate diagnosis, and consequent treatment.

# Sounds of Silence

## *Community Impact*

O'Hara (2003) suggests that, while a diagnosis of learning disability cuts across racial, religious or cultural boundaries, attitudes to people with learning disabilities have strong socio-ethnic variations. As recently as 1971, women with learning disabilities were mandatorily sterilised and forbidden to marry in twenty-four US states. In contrast, in some Bengali communities, marriage for an adult with a learning disability may be seen as offering a person protection after the death of their own parents. The socioeconomic status of black and ethnic minority [BEM] people in twenty-first century Britain is as diverse as for any other group, but statistically, it is claimed that the prevalence of learning disability among South Asian communities is three times that of levels among the general population (DH 2001). This has been linked to inequalities of healthcare (Emerson 1997). Based on these statistics, Gill and Badger (2007) calculate that, given there are around three million BEM people in England, around sixty thousand people from BEM communities will seek healthcare at some stage in their lives. Reporting to the Department of Health [DH], Mir et al (DH 2001) believe that poor and inappropriate communication are contributory factors, not only to the prevalence of learning disability, but to the limited knowledge of, and access to, services which might be able to help the individuals concerned.

It is also apparent that women with learning disabilities, who are, additionally, members of any ethnic minority, may face *triple jeopardy*, due to their ethnicity, disability, and gender (DH 2001, 12):

> people with learning difficulties from a minority ethnic community experienced simultaneous disadvantage in relation to race, impairment and, for women, gender.

Often, not only are treatment and interaction with medical professionals inequitable, but therapies suggested by medical professionals may be inappropriate to the individual, as they may require participation in mixed-gender activities, or might, in other ways, conflict with cultural or religious beliefs. These issues are further complicated when an interpreter is used, whether a family member, or one provided by an advocacy service. The interpreter needs to be briefed carefully to ensure that communication is not hindered by the interpreter's own cultural beliefs, which may, for example, preclude the discussion of sexuality (Nadirshaw 1997; Ravel 1996; Shah 1992). Further, the National Autistic Society's report, *Missing Out* (Corbett and Perepa 2007), notes that in some languages there is no word for autism, and this can lead to confusion for families if it is translated as 'mental health' or 'learning disability' instead. Even a skilled and culturally sensitive interpreter can disempower the patient, and their family members and carers, perhaps preventing them from seeking help from appropriate services in the future.

The health of people with learning disabilities is often significantly poorer than that of the rest of the UK population generally. In addition, the incidence of co-existing conditions in many people with learning disabilities is often higher (Elliott et al 2003; Corbett 2007). This means that the needs of PLDs may have a more significant impact on communities, and mainstream community health services, following the closure of long-stay institutions (DH 2001). Like the rest of the UK population, people with learning disabilities are generally living longer. This increases the need for equitable access to healthcare (DH 2001).

## Co-existing Medical Conditions

The National Autistic Society reported in 2010 that it is often difficult, if not impossible, to encourage people with autistic spectrum disorders to attend routine medical examinations and dental appointments. Further, there are low statistics for people with learning disabilities seeking and undergoing routine health checks for breast cancer (Hermon et al 2001), and cervical cancer (Pearson et al 1998). Statistically, these findings correlate directly with the incidence of cancers and oral diseases, which occur less frequently in members of the general population who do not have this personal barrier to preventative examinations. Further, there is increasing statistical evidence that people with learning disabilities have a higher rate of co-existing health issues, including gastro-intestinal cancer (Cooke 1997, Jancar 1990). Moreover, in comparison with the general population, PLDs are three times more likely to have schizophrenia (Doody et al 1998) alongside neuro-typical prevalence of mental health issues, anxiety, depression, and challenging behaviours (Emerson 2003). Children with Down's syndrome are at a particularly high risk of leukaemia and congenital heart problems (Brookes and Alberman 1996). Additionally, those with Down's syndrome are at a particularly high risk of developing dementia, with an onset age of 30-40 years younger than the general population (Holland et al 1998).

## Contaminated Consent

The *Mental Capacity Act* (2009) provides a statutory framework for people who may not be able to make their own decisions, for example because of learning difficulties, brain trauma, mental health problems, or a combination of these. There is a wide range of practices for determining mental capacity for the purposes of giving consent (Nicholson et al 2008; Javed and Afzal 2009), and innovative work has been carried out in this area by Suzanne Conboy-Hill. Conboy-Hill (2006) has developed a cognitive interview method, evolved from techniques used by police to interview child victims of abuse. Her research has identified that, during questioning to assess mental capacity, PLDs are likely to react in ways that make their responses unreliable. They may be susceptible to suggestion, or to acquiescence, may exhibit global memory difficulties, may be dependent on external cues, or may exhibit communication difficulties. In particular, they are prone to answer in the affirmative, even when they have not understood the question; to choose the second of two choices, as they are more likely to remember more recent information better; and to be easily influenced by leading questions. Unless great care is taken by the person attempting to take consent, there is a high likelihood of contaminated and inaccurate reports, which can compromise the best interests of the patient.

Conboy-Hill's cognitive interview method increases the probability of the best interests of patients being upheld, but it is slow, time-consuming, and requires training. We hope that, by raising postgraduate doctors' awareness of how they support patients with learning disabilities, our workshops will encourage them to engage with methods such as this process for obtaining consent, perhaps with assistance from other experienced health professionals, as one way of improving patient safety.

## Breaking Silence

Although all of the National Curriculum Frameworks [NCFs] for PGME include professionalism (see Chapter 11) and communication, they do not specifically take into account working with PLDs. However, as part of my work on the KSS Qualified Education Supervisor Programme [QESP] (see Chapter 4), I have discussed with hospital consultants their experiences of supporting PLDs. Their general reaction has been interest in learning how to improve their own interactions, recognition that this is an important practical area of learning for postgraduate doctors, but also concern about the relative scarcity of good learning materials.

A search of KSS Library and Knowledge Services [LKS] for books and articles on working with PLDs confirmed the anecdotal view of the scarcity of resources. Some LEPs had no publications immediately available, while others had up to ten publications, aimed mainly at non-medical health professionals. Only one book (*Health Care Provision and People with Learning Disabilities* by Jo Corbett 2007) appeared on shelves at the majority of LEPs. An immediate step was for KSS LKS to ensure that, in future, all LEPs will have a standard set of current materials; a second step was for the Education Department to develop additional, specialist materials. These materials are targeted at Foundation but are, of course, applicable to all grades and specialties.

### *Project Development*

The original project team drew on the knowledge, qualities, and skills of several members of the KSS Deanery's Education team, a professional services co-ordinator, who is also an anthropologist, and an external consultant, Catherine Filby, who contributed the voice of the carer, gained from years of caring for her sister (C) above, who has learning disabilities. As a team, we agreed that the patients' voices would be represented through filmed conversations with them.

One of the starting points for programme development was a commissioned short report entitled *Patients with Learning Disabilities from a Carer's Perspective* (Filby 2009), which combined the writer's and other people's experiences of accompanying PLDs to healthcare appointments. It described both positive and negative experiences, such as a thoughtful optician, who took extra time with a service user who had never been for an eye test before, and who did not understand instructions. This experience led to the service user now feeling comfortable attending optician appointments unaccompanied. A contrast was provided by an account of a gynaecologist, who informed a service user during a smear test that she should have her womb removed, because she was a woman with intellectual disabilities. On this occasion, support from the carer enabled the service user to complain, and a referral to a different consultant was made.

A further starting point was to define and agree on an appropriate term for the patients whose needs we were to consider. In the *Valuing People* white paper, learning disability is defined as:

> a condition which includes the presence of a significantly reduced ability to understand new or complex information or to learn new skills (impaired intelligence) with a reduced ability to cope independently (impaired social functioning). These must have started before adulthood and have a lasting effect on development (DH 2009, 14).

We researched and discussed a range of possibilities: 'vulnerable patients', 'patients with mental health issues', 'patients with intellectual disabilities', 'patients with special needs'. Eventually we agreed on the term 'patients with learning disabilities'. In a medical setting, all patients have special needs and are vulnerable. While some people prefer 'learning difficulties', this can lead to confusion, as it is also used in educational settings to describe conditions such as dyslexia. The term 'learning disabilities' has been used in the UK since the early 1990s, and since it appears in current literature from organisations such as the DH, Mencap, and the Royal College of Nursing, we felt that this term might offer an important access route to track resources and support.

## *Workshop Format*

A key concern was to develop a format that would enable postgraduate doctors to use it as the basis for developing their practice in the complex, problematic, real-life world of clinical care. As a matter of good educational practice, the workshop would require a participative manner of learning. At the same time, we recognised that care for PLDs is an emergent curriculum area for PGME, with relatively little specialist, in-depth literature. Accordingly, we would require a high level of willingness to engage from participants.

An early decision was to focus on obtaining consent. We wanted to encourage participants to recognise and discuss the different voices present in an interaction with PLDs, and to reflect on how they could best uphold their patient's best interests. We were very clear that the workshop would have to be grounded in practice, discussion, and reflection, and believed that reductionist approaches, such as 'ten top tips for managing patients with learning disabilities', had little to offer of practical value. Instead, we set out to develop an intellectually safe workshop environment, which would enable participants to explore their perceptions of learning disability.

Pragmatically, we discovered that it was necessary to timetable the workshop to take place during a timetabled teaching session, if it was to attract enough participants to form a viable group. Accordingly, after some experimentation, we decided not to offer the workshop to Foundation Year One [F1] doctors, unless that was requested specifically by an LEP. Our experience was that Foundation Year Two [F2] was the most successful location in the Foundation curriculum for the workshop.

## Early Findings

It was noticeable that some participants expected the workshop to be run on the 'banking approach' (Freire 1972), in which they would passively receive deposits of information. Some appeared disappointed to find that the workshop concentrated on challenging perceptions and attitudes, and on developing interaction and communication. A very few participants felt that there was nothing to discuss, with one person commenting, 'You don't waste time, you just knock them out with tranquillisers, and do whatever you need to do'. However, the majority of participants engage with interest and, in particular, discussion of their own personal experiences with PLDs catalyses general discussion and debate. Film clips of conversations with PLDs are equally effective, since participants are able to pick out segments from the clips, and discuss the statements made by the speakers. One participant reflected that it 'put a human face' on the label 'learning disabilities'. In particular, the film clip of (A), an individual close to participants' own ages, and with an acquired learning disability, not a congenital one, has the ability to silence workshop participants, and encourages them to question their perceptions of PLDs.

At the end of the workshop, participants complete blank-sheet evaluations to encourage free-form feedback. Comments have included:

> Very informative, friendly and excellent speaker, was interactive
> A video of good communication style
> Interesting, stimulated thought
> Very useful session as currently very limited exposure to communicating and managing parents with learning disabilities
> Session is a really important topic, very relevant
> Good examples on taking time to understand more about the patient's perceptions of doctors and the importance of careful discharge planning

## Next Steps

We shall continue to provide our workshop on PLDs to KSS LEPs, as a minimum curriculum entitlement for PGME. However, it is clear that it is relevant to other healthcare professionals as well, and we have already taught it to sixty pre-registration pharmacists, while one LEP wishes to extend it to all of its clinical workforce. Certainly, we view work with PLDs as an important part of the KSS patient-safety agenda, and as fundamental to developing professionalism.

Accompanying this work, we hope that LEPs will also improve access to healthcare through 'quick-fixes', such as improving access to healthcare through better signage, easy-to-read versions of healthcare information, health-facilitation planning, and patient passports. However, these are clearly not an alternative to equipping doctors with the confidence and skills to work more effectively with PLDs.

Finally, of course our PLD project cannot address the way society as a whole perceives people with a learning disability. However, every occasion which challenges conventional thinking about how we interact with people with learning disabilities may be a small step towards their more equitable treatment. As Martin Luther King (1963) said in his *A Time to Break Silence* speech: 'Our lives begin to end the day we become silent about things which matter'.

# References

Astor, R. 2001. Detecting Pain in People with Profound Learning Disabilities, *Nursing Times*. Oct 4-10. 97. 40: 38-9.

Brookes, M. E. and E. Alberman. 1996. Early Mortality and Morbidity in Children with Down's Syndrome Diagnosed in Two Regional Health Authorities in 1988. *Journal of Medical Screening* 3: 7-11.

Conboy-Hill, S. 2006. Vulnerable Adults; Assessing Capacity to Consent, *Clinical Psychology Forum* 158: 19-23.

Cooke, L. B. 1997. Cancer and Learning Disability, *Journal of Intellectual Disability Research*. 41. 4: 312–316.

Cooper, A. M. 1988. *Healthcare and the Autism spectrum: A Guide for Health Professionals*. London: Jessica Kingsley.

Corbett, C. and P. Perepa. 2007. *Missing Out*. National Autistic Society: London.

Corbett, J. 2007. *Health Care Provision and People with Learning Disabilities*. Chichester: Wiley.

Davis, B. and W. G. Schunick. 2002. *Dangerous Encounters – Avoiding Perilous Situations with Autism*. London: Jessica Kingsley.

Department of Health. 2001. *Learning Difficulties and Ethnicity*. Report by Mir, G., A. Nocon, W. Ahmad and L. Jones. London: DH.

Department of Health. 2008. *Healthcare for All*. [Michael Report]. London: DH.

Department of Health. 2009. *Valuing People: A New Three-Year Strategy for People with Learning Difficulties*. London: DH.

Doody, G. A., M. Gotz, E. C. Johnstone, C. D. Frith.and D. G. Cunningham Owens. 1998. Theory of Mind and Psychoses, *Psychological Medicine* 28. 2: 397-405. Cambridge: University Press.

Elliott, J., C. Hatton and E. Emerson. 2003. The Health of People with Learning Disabilities in the UK: Evidence and Implications for the NHS, *Journal of Integrated Care*. 11. 3: 7-9.

Emerson, E. 1997. Is there an Increased Prevalence of Severe Learning Disabilities among British Asians? *Ethnicity and Health*, 2: 317-321.

Emerson, E. 2003. Prevalence of Psychiatric Disorders in Children and Adolescents With and Without Intellectual Disability. *Journal of Intellectual Disability Research*. 47. 1: 51-58.

Emerson, E. and C. Hatton. 2004. *Estimating Future Need/Demand for Supports for People with Learning Disabilities in England*. http://www.lancs.ac.uk/shm/dhr/research/learning/download/futureneed.pdf. (accessed 28 January 2011).

Freire, P. 1972. *Pedagogy of the Oppressed*. Translated by Myra Bergman Ramos. Harmondsworth: Penguin.

Gill, R., and J. Badger. 2007. The Concept of Advocacy and Culturally and Ethnically Diverse Communities, *British Institute of Learning Disabilities*, unpublished paper.

Hermon, C., E. Alberman, V. Beral and A. J. Swerdlow. 2001. Mortality and cancer incidence in persons with Down's syndrome, their parents and siblings. *Annals of Human Genetics* 65: 167-176.

Holland, A. J. 2000. Ageing and learning disability. *British Journal of Psychiatry* 176: 26-31.

Holland, A. J., J. Hon, F. A. Huppert, S. Stevens and P. Watson. 1998. Population-based study of the prevalence and presentation of dementia in adults with Down's syndrome. *British Journal of Psychiatry* 172: 493-498.

Jackson, L. 2002. *Freaks, Geeks and Asperger Syndrome*: A User Guide to Adolescence. London: Jessica Kingsley.

Jancar, J. 1990. Cancer and mental handicap: a further study. *British Journal of Psychiatry* 156: 531-533.

Javed, A. and M. Afzal. 2009. Assessing Mental Capacity, *Pakistan Journal of Medical Sciences* 25 (3): 516-519.

Jopp, D. A. and C. B. Keys. 2001. Diagnostic Overshadowing Reviewed and Reconsidered, *American Journal on Mental Retardation*: 106, (5): 416-433.

Kerr, D. 2007. *Understanding learning disability and dementia: Developing effective interventions*. London: Jessica Kingsley.

King, M. L. *A Time to Break Silence*. 28 August 1963. http://www.americanrhetoric.com/speeches/mlkatimetobreaksilence.htm. (accessed 30 January 2011).

Local Government Ombudsman and Parliamentary and Health Service Ombudsman. 2009. *Six Lives: the provision of public services to people with learning disabilities*. Second Report. London: HMSO.

Mason, J. and K. Scior. 2004. Diagnostic overshadowing' amongst clinicians working with people with intellectual disabilities in the UK. *Journal of Applied Research in Intellectual Disabilities* 17 (2): 85-90.

McArdle, E. 2001. Communication Impairment and Stigma. *In Stigma and Social Exclusion in Healthcare, eds*. T. Mason, C. Watkins, C. Carlisle and E. Whitehead. London: Routledge.

Mencap. 2007. *Death by Indifference*. London: Mencap.

Nadirshaw, Z. 1997. Cultural Issues. In *Adults with Learning Disabilities: Approach for Health Professionals, eds*. J. O'Hara and A. Sperlinger: 139-153. Chichester: John Wiley.

National Aphasia Association *What is Aphasia?* http://www.aphasia.org/Aphasia%20Facts/aphasia_facts.html. (accessed 17 January 2011).

Nicholson, T. R. J., W. Cutter and M. Hotopf. 2008. Assessing Mental Capacity: the Mental Capacity Act, *BMJ*, 336:322 (10): 1136.

O'Hara, J. 2003. Learning Disabilities and Ethnicity: Achieving Cultural Competence. *Advances in Psychiatric Treatment* 9: 166-176.

Pearson, V., C. Davis, C. Ruoff and J. Dyer. 1998. Only One Quarter of Women with Learning Disability in Exeter Have Cervical Screening. *BMJ* 316: 1979.

Ravel, H. 1996. A Systemic Perspective on Working with Interpreters. *Clinical Child Psychology and Psychiatry* 1: 29-43.

Royal College of Psychiatrists 2010. *Fair Deal for Mental Health Campaign*. http://www.rcpsych.ac.uk/campaigns/fairdeal.aspx. (accessed 30 January 2011)

Sainsbury, C. 2000. *Martin in the Playground: Understanding the Schoolchild with Asperger's Syndrome*. England: Lucky Duck Publishing.

Shah, R. 1992 (revised edition 1995). *The Silent Majority: Children with Disabilities in Asian Families*. London: National Children's Bureau.

# Managing Medical Careers in a Changing World

Traditionally, a career in medicine has been viewed as a mark of prestige and success. While this is still true, the recent sweeping changes to medical career pathways and healthcare in the UK have removed some of the old certainties, necessitating new thought and new support structures. The Modernising Medical Careers [MMC] initiative of 2007 sought to improve patient care through reforms to postgraduate medical education [PGME]. This has resulted in a need to provide medical students and postgraduate doctors with information, resources, and career support to assist them in career management and in navigating their way through the new medical career pathways.

Postgraduate doctors work within the National Health Service [NHS] as employees, while at the same time being educated under the auspices of Postgraduate Medical Deaneries [Deaneries]. There is a need, therefore, to prepare these doctors to meet the requirements of the UK's healthcare service, while also taking into account their own career expectations and development as 'whole' individuals. In many cases, contemporary postgraduate doctors have found it challenging to make career choices earlier in their PGME than they were planning to do when they first entered medical school. At the same time, medical career pathways continue to be subject to changes resulting from demographic factors, advances in technology, and increased public expectations of the NHS. This chapter considers how medical careers in these changing contexts can be understood and managed within the medical profession, from both an individual and an organisational perspective.

## Careers: Definitions and Terminology

A wide range of terminology is used within the careers field. The term 'career' itself, in common use in the early 1800s, became defined in a number of different ways as its usage increased. Hall (1976) uses the concept of 'career' to include ideas such as advancement, profession, a lifelong sequence of jobs and a sequence of role-related experiences. Arnold (1997, 16) defines career as 'The sequence of employment related positions, roles, activities and experiences encountered by a person'. This definition is broader, although it does not explicitly acknowledge the internal and external influences on a person's career. More recently, Watts (1999, 22) suggests the need to redefine the word 'career', as it no longer represents a neat progression upwards through a hierarchy. He redefines 'career' as 'the individual's lifelong progression in learning and in work' – a definition particularly relevant to the interlinked themes of service and learning within contemporary medical careers, as postgraduate doctors are at once employed in NHS organisations and engaged in education.

Careers professionals who work with undergraduates and postgraduates, are familiar with the following definitions (DENI 2009, 4):

> **Careers Information** provides access to up-to-date impartial labour market information and information relating to educational and training opportunities, to inform career planning and management.

> **Careers Advice and Guidance** is the provision of impartial, learner / client-centered advice and guidance, to assist in making appropriate career decisions and choices which are informed and well thought through. It enables people to apply their knowledge, understanding, skills and experiences to manage their career and make informed decisions about their education, training or employment.

Within organisations, people who work with individuals often refer to terms such as 'career development' and 'career management' (Cedefop 2008). Career professionals who work with individuals to provide career information, advice, and guidance are seen as independent, and it is the individual who gains benefit from their support. However, career development and management within an organisational context is often aimed at benefiting both the individual and the organisation itself. Potentially, this can lead to tension if the needs of the organisation are prioritised above those of the individual. However, a large-scale investigation by Hirsh et al (2001), involving a consortium of employers, identified that the provision of career support from within an organisation was seen as beneficial by the recipients, even though it was provided by their employer.

In 2006, Kent, Surrey and Sussex Postgraduate Medical Deanery [KSS] Education Department commissioned Caroline Elton to develop a careers support model which could be used with postgraduate doctors on the Foundation Programme [Foundation]. Elton (2006) recognised the importance of putting in place a structure that was underpinned by a theoretical model of career decision making, and that also recognised the roles that Local Education Providers [LEPs] and Deanery-based staff have in providing effective career support. This chapter draws on the work carried out by Elton (2006) and focuses on the need to provide career support to postgraduate doctors in Foundation, Core Specialty Training [CST], and Higher Specialty Training [HST]. The main aim of the KSS career support model is to increase the capacity of postgraduate doctors to develop their own career management skills, and also to support the development of their teachers (usually Educational Supervisors or Training Programme Directors [TPDs]) in providing career support in our LEPs.

## Changing Professional and Career Pathways

The MMC programme was initiated with the aim of improving patient care by modernising and focusing the career structure of postgraduate doctors, which necessitated extensive reform of PGME. The reforms introduced a new career pathway, which included Foundation Year One [F1] and Year Two [F2] and a range of CST and HST Programmes. Foundation replaced the first two years of clinical practice for medical graduates, which formerly comprised the Pre-Registration House Officer [PRHO] year and the first year of the Senior House Officer [SHO] grade. CST and HST were designed to follow on from Foundation (see Figure 1). Specialty training programmes are usually offered either as 'run-through training', often referred to as 'coupled' (e.g. Paediatrics and General Practice), or 'uncoupled' (see Figure 1). Uncoupled training normally comprises CST for two to three years, followed by competitive entry to HST for a period of four to six years. Examples of uncoupled specialties include all Medical specialties, Anaesthetics, and Psychiatry.

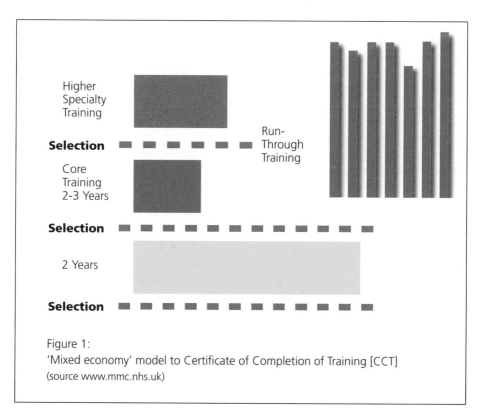

Figure 1:
'Mixed economy' model to Certificate of Completion of Training [CCT]
(source www.mmc.nhs.uk)

The Department of Health [DH] recognised that doctors in Foundation would need access to high-quality assistance in planning their careers. One of the eighteen key principles that underpin MMC states that: 'Rigorous counselling and career advice should be available throughout training' (MMC 2003, 3). Foundation itself reflects this intention: it has both an operational framework and a curriculum supported by a portfolio, in which every Foundation doctor is expected to record their educational achievements and the results of their assessments. A section of the portfolio is available to record thoughts on possible career choices. Recent updates to these documents have included changes to the operational framework and to the curriculum, and these will further encourage the development of career choice and decision making by Foundation doctors.

While the portfolio and curriculum certainly help to make clear the need to plan ahead, postgraduate doctors have continued to express concerns about their having to make career choices at an earlier stage than was required under the 'old system'. In some cases, these have been serious enough to result in a desire to leave medicine. Pre-MMC, data from the Higher Education Funding Council for England [HEFCE], supported by British Medical Association [BMA] Cohort Study 1995-2005, suggest that 0.6 – 1% of medical graduates were not in PRHO posts six months after graduation: the majority of them were working in other sectors. The ninth report from this BMA cohort study found that 7% of the cohort had left the UK medical workforce. The most common reasons stated for leaving medicine as a career were dissatisfaction with medicine, the attraction of other careers and working conditions and pay in the NHS.

After the MMC reforms were implemented, much work was carried out by Deaneries to ensure that career support was in place, to manage the expectations of postgraduate doctors, and to provide them with the skills to manage their own careers. Foundation provided a number of key documents to help this process, including *The Rough Guide to Foundation* and the learning portfolio. Foundation's intention was that postgraduate doctors should be responsible for their own learning and career progression, supported by Foundation Schools and teachers in LEPs. Deanery and Foundation School efforts have been focused on encouraging postgraduate doctors to continue their medical careers; so far, little research has been carried out into the decision-making process itself, or into the factors that influence postgraduate doctors' decisions to leave clinical practice.

One study does provide some broad indications of these factors: when Moss et al (2004) from the UK Medical Careers Group surveyed postgraduate doctors by questionnaire to ascertain their reasons for considering leaving UK medicine, 1,047 out of 1,326 respondents indicated they would stay in medicine, but not necessarily in the UK. Of 279 postgraduate doctors considering leaving medicine, 72% gave reasons related to UK working conditions, 23% gave reasons associated with life-style choices and the remainder reported positive interest in a different career. However, this study did not examine the career support or decision-making processes employed. A year later, Turner et al (2005) reported that postgraduate doctors take into account quality-of-life issues and long-term career prospects when making long-term career decisions.

As the MMC reforms began to take effect, public interest and strongly voiced concerns within the medical profession led to an independent DH inquiry, which culminated in the Tooke Report (2007). Tooke recognised the need for accurate data on career aspirations and choices, and advised that medical schools should play a greater role in providing careers advice. The Report suggested that medical schools should: provide information in their prospectuses about career destinations and competition ratios; offer selective components to allow experiences in discrete specialties; and provide formal personalised advice / mentoring. A further recommendation was that Postgraduate Medical Deans should have 'strong accountability links to medical schools as well as SHAs' which would 'improve links with major academic expertise and . . . facilitate the educational continuum from student to continuing professional development' (Tooke 2007, 111). The role Deaneries might play in providing career support was not mentioned in the Report. That Report was followed by the DH's *NHS Next Stage Review* and the Darzi Report (2008, 14), *High Quality Care for All*, which identified the need for 'a clear focus on improving the quality of NHS education and training'. The provision of careers information, advice, and guidance to doctors and particularly to postgraduate doctors will continue to be challenged by changes to medical career pathways as the recommendations from both the Tooke and the Darzi Reports are implemented.

At an operational level, careers advisers working with medical schools and in Deaneries are continuing to develop the services they provide for medical students and for postgraduate doctors. The Medical Schools Council is also providing information on careers. My own experience in KSS took as its starting point the need to embed careers in the Foundation curriculum, producing a range of interventions and resources to support both teachers and postgraduate doctors.

## New Structures and New Forms of Support

Many consultants who supervise postgraduate doctors have raised concerns about how best to support and advise them. They feel that the advice that they were given when they were postgraduate doctors themselves no longer makes sense, and they find the new career system unclear. In the context of these rapid and far-reaching changes, previous models of career support required a radical rethink. Since the late 1990s, a number of studies such as Jackson et al (2003), have shown a continuing and increasing need to develop and augment the careers advice available for doctors at all stages of their careers. Both the BMA and the UK Medical Careers Group carry out extensive cohort studies into career choice and career progression in medicine. The BMA has followed up two cohorts of doctors – cohort one of 545 doctors who graduated in 1995 and cohort two of 435 doctors who graduated in 2006. The BMA's 2003 report *Signposting Medical Careers for Doctors* made eight key recommendations, one of which was that 'further research is needed to test the effectiveness of the various methods of delivering careers advice' (BMA 2003, 2).

The third report of the BMA's cohort study of the medical graduates of 2006 states that six in ten cohort doctors prefer a career in medicine and three in ten prefer a career in General Practice. The most recent review of medical workforce needs (Darzi 2008) suggests that the changing requirements of the NHS and demographic shifts indicate the need for more general practitioners [GPs] and fewer hospital specialties. The doctors in the BMA's 2006 cohort study were surveyed in 2009 at the end of F2, and fewer than 5% of them were undecided about their career option. However, even this level of indecision suggested a need for further guidance as well as support for those people who may not get into their first choice specialty. The tenth report of the BMA's cohort study of 1995-2005 medical graduates proposed that appropriate measures should be put in place to ensure that medical education includes the necessary subject material and processes to prepare doctors for a career in modern medicine. This report also went on to suggest that a mentoring scheme might be introduced at medical school and that the practice of mentoring might be continued throughout a doctor's career, particularly in the early stages, to provide career guidance. In more recent work, Taylor et al (2008) identified that the need for careers advice applies not just to postgraduate doctors. Their survey of career-grade doctors highlighted the need for career development on a lifelong basis. However, concerns were raised by respondents about its availability, about the time it might take, about impartiality and about confidentiality. The issue of confidentiality is of prime importance, and is taken into consideration by the KSS approach to the provision of career support.

## The Organisation and the Individual

In common with some other professions, postgraduate doctors are employees as well as learners. A Cedefop Report (2008, 33) recognises that tensions are inherent in employer-led career support schemes. It indicates that many organisations have no clear processes for career development. Further, where it does exist, career development at work can often lack clear objectives for employees, and may result in self-help strategies that are difficult to implement. Employees may also be suspicious of employers' motives. The Cedefop Report recognised an increasing use of the internet and a blurring of the boundaries between career support and recruitment activities, peer support, and the development of virtual community websites. It stressed the importance of individuals being able to acquire for themselves the skills necessary for successful career management. The Report concluded that much remains to be done to provide fully effective career development to people in organisations. Clearly, for such schemes to succeed, the needs of both the individual and the organisation should be recognised and acknowledged. These are all issues that we have attempted to address in devising a career-support model for KSS.

## Career Management in Context: the KSS Approach

Building on the requirements set out by MMC, Deaneries responded in different ways to the requirement to provide career support to Foundation doctors. At KSS, Caroline Elton carried out a career-implementation project with the overall aim of identifying options for the efficient and effective provision of support for career planning for Foundation doctors. In her Report (Elton 2006), she presented a model underpinned by two key elements: a four-stage career-planning framework, which is widely used in the provision of careers advice in Education (see Figure 2) and a three-tier support model (see Figure 3).

Elton (2006) explored what a 'gold standard' career support service would look like, and reviewed both the career-management model proposed by MMC and the provision made by other Deaneries. The four-stage framework outlined in Figure 2 is well known in the career-management area and is intended to help providers of one-to-one career-support work. It can be used flexibly to meet individual needs.

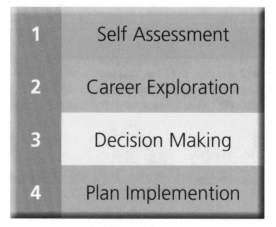

Figure 2: Four-stage career-planning framework
Source: www.medicalcareers.nhs.uk

The second key aspect of Elton's Report was the recommendation that most of the career support required by Foundation doctors should be provided at LEP level. In KSS we adopted a three-tier model for postgraduate doctors in Foundation (Elton 2006). At LEP level, we proposed that individual postgraduate doctors should discuss their career aspirations and plans during regular meetings with their Educational Supervisors, and that they should include information about career planning in their Foundation portfolios. Medical Education Managers [MEMs], Library and Knowledge Services [LKS] staff, and support staff working in the LEP's education centre were key players in LEP-based support of this kind. Furthermore, an additional role, entitled 'Faculty Career Lead' was created. This role has been operating successfully for some time and is usually carried out by a Foundation Educational Supervisor or TPD. The Faculty Career Lead plays an important part in educational governance for the LEP, and sits on the Local Faculty Group [LFG] for Foundation. The role of LFGs is described in Chapters 1 and 3.

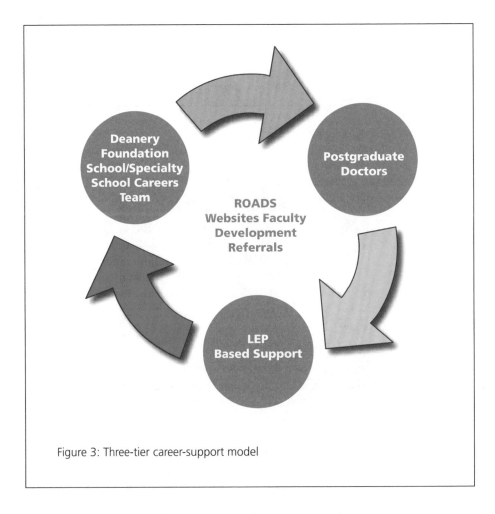

Figure 3: Three-tier career-support model

## Implementing the Three-Tier Model

When I joined KSS in 2006, the career-support project was moving into its implementation phase. The first activity was to develop staff in LEPs to provide career support to Foundation doctors. We also hoped at this stage to identify people who would take on the Faculty Career Lead role in LEPs. Caroline Elton is a registered occupational psychologist and has had extensive experience of working as a Consultant Education Adviser [CEA] at KSS on the Certificate in Teaching as well as with a wide range of clients in her own career-counselling practice. As I have experience working as a career coach in a large corporate organisation, our combined understanding of what comprises good career support has enabled us to help people think about the choices they face at important transition points in their careers.

Initial development for staff in LEPs took the form of a conference attended by over a hundred people. We provided a variety of presentations and workshops, including an outline of the four-stage career-planning framework and sessions on interests, values, decision making and interviews. A subsequent workshop for Faculty Career Leads included further materials that had been developed to help postgraduate doctors apply for specialty programmes. This workshop also included skill development in managing career conversations. After the workshop a range of resources was devised, including plans for further workshops that LEPs could run themselves for F1 and F2 doctors. These resources were used as the basis for producing *The ROADS to Success* [ROADS], a career-planning guide for medical students, Foundation doctors, and their Educational Supervisors.

While we were working on materials at KSS to help support Foundation doctors with their career decisions, the MMC programme continued to develop further with the implementation of specialty training programmes and the introduction of new recruitment methods and timescales. The timing of career decisions by postgraduate doctors became important for those who wished to progress from Foundation to CST. Recruitment into CST commenced in December 2009, with postgraduate doctors actually taking up their appointments in August 2010 or later, depending on the specialty. Effectively, postgraduate doctors now needed to make their career choices part-way through F2. In 2006 it was certainly the case that not all medical schools provided career support, and it was clear that both medical students and postgraduate doctors would benefit from information and resources to help them bridge the gap between medical school and PGME. In KSS, this came in the form of ROADS.

## Developing ROADS

The first edition of ROADS was published by KSS in 2007 and the book is currently in its third edition (Elton and Reid 2010). It is aimed both at individuals facing particular career choices and challenges and at their Educational Supervisors, and includes guidance on running both one-to-one and group career-support sessions. There are sections on each of the four stages in the career-planning framework, a section for Educational Supervisors, and appendices which include plans for workshops for F1 and F2 doctors.

The book is informed by the work of a number of writers including Hirsh et al (2001), Krieshok et al (2009), and Borges and Savickas (2002). Hirsh et al (2001) considered organisational approaches to career provision and highlighted the importance of a shared framework to be used by the provider and recipient of career support, and this recommendation has been incorporated into ROADS. The tools and resources to aid specialty choice were the subject of an extensive literature review carried out by Borges and Savickas (2002). Their findings suggested that the Myers Briggs Type Indicator (Borges and Savickas 2002) was the most commonly used psychometric instrument to support medical specialty choice. We therefore included an extensive section on the use of psychometric instruments to support career planning for doctors.

## Web-based Resources

Some of the initial careers resources originally written for LEP training events were also made available on the internet, namely on the KSS careers website, which has continued to develop (it can be viewed at http://www.kssDeanery.org/careers). The importance of providing quality information over the internet is well recognised (Offer and Sampson 1999 and Oliver and Whiston 2000). Offer and Sampson suggested the need for a 'self-diagnostic' package, perhaps linking the results to other specific kite-marked sites. While the KSS careers site adopted this second suggestion to a limited extent, by 2007 there was widespread interest in utilising the materials developed by the Association of American Medical Colleges [AAMC] Careers in Medicine Programme. This had been supported by Elton (2006) in her Report for KSS.

In the USA, medicine is studied not as an undergraduate subject but at a postgraduate level after individuals have completed a first degree in another subject. The American medical degree is usually taken over four years, and AAMC has developed an extensive careers programme (www.aamc.org/careersinmedicine) to aid students in their fourth year at medical school to choose their specialty. Despite the differences in duration and timing, the American programme is nevertheless directly relevant to F2. At the instigation of the Head of Education at KSS, Professor Playdon, a national project was proposed and supported by MMC to set up a NHS Medical Careers website (www.medicalcareers.nhs.uk) based on the licensing of materials from AAMC. KSS was asked to take over further development and management of the site in 2008.

The site aims to address the increasing need for medical careers advice, information, and resources. Patel et al (2008, 231) reported that 'medical students prefer computer-based technology and rapidly adapt to new resources on the web because of its availability, ease of use and speed in retrieving relevant information'. The site has a wide user base: medical students, postgraduate doctors, teachers, and support staff. It provides an integrated approach to career provision, with the intention of providing a single location for information on medical specialties, including case studies and podcasts, workforce information and interactive tools to support career planning. KSS has continued to extend the site by developing its platform, adding new content and increasingly making use of podcasts and more personalised information, such as case studies, in response to requests from the site's focus group and users.

## Faculty Development

When the KSS three-tier model was first implemented, development sessions were provided for Faculty Career Leads. However, a large number of Educational Supervisors and TPDs in KSS were interested in learning more. Initially the careers team developed a one-day career-support workshop, including an overview of the four-stage framework and information and resources for use when working with individuals. This workshop is run six times a year and is well attended. It forms a useful follow-on to KSS's Qualified Educational Supervisor Programme [QESP], since it develops the careers aspects that are introduced in QESP Part 2 (see Chapter 4 of this book).

Caroline Elton (2006) proposed that there should be research into the provision of a Postgraduate Certificate in career planning, specifically to support doctors and others involved in medical education. This research was carried out, and the KSS Education Department and careers team developed a Postgraduate Certificate in Managing Medical Careers which was validated in 2007 through the University of Brighton. The course comprises three modules: working with individuals; working with groups; and working in an organisation. It introduces participants to career theory and to educational theory, including concepts such as communities of practice, change management, and leadership, all in the context of medical education and the medical career pathway. The first cohort for the Postgraduate Certificate commenced in January 2008 and is currently in its third year. The course participants are all involved in medical education and careers provision in the UK, and include people who have Deanery and LEP management roles in medical education. More recently, KSS has developed a progression route from the Postgraduate Certificate to a Postgraduate Diploma and to the degree of Master of Arts [MA], which we have validated through the Institute of Postgraduate Medicine at Brighton and Sussex Medical School. The new Postgraduate Diploma commenced in January 2011 and the Masters year is planned to commence in 2012. The Diploma year will build on the Certificate and include modules on advanced guidance skills, work and well-being, and research methods with the MA year focusing on a dissertation and a portfolio.

## Working with Postgraduate Doctors

The KSS careers team regularly supports the work of KSS LEPs by running workshops for F1 and F2 doctors. The F1 workshops generally concentrate on introducing the career-planning framework and the first two stages: self-assessment and career exploration. Workshops for

F2s usually focus on stages three and four: decision making and plan implementation. In addition, they provide specific information and resources about the recruitment process for specialty programmes. The team also runs specific workshops for F2s on applications and interviews, and team members attend the specialty recruitment evenings arranged by the KSS Specialty Workforce team. This can make for a busy time in the Autumn as the careers team also attends a number of careers fairs and events around the country, such as the two main BMJ careers fairs.

Another recent development is a pilot project to provide drop-in sessions with a careers adviser for Foundation doctors. LEPs have taken up the offer and provided a confidential space in their Education Centres for a careers adviser to see up to six people a day in half-hour slots. Foundation doctors have made use of these slots to explore a wide range of issues with an adviser. This pilot project was subsequently extended to other KSS LEPs from Autumn 2010.

The careers team also supports induction events provided by the KSS Specialty Schools and provides an overview of career planning. This work ensures that the careers team is ideally placed to provide well-informed workshops for F2 doctors, and to support KSS specialty recruitment evenings.

At a national level, the KSS careers team has representatives on the committee of the Association of Graduate Careers Advisory Services / Medical Careers Advisers' Network [MCAN] and the National Educational Advisers' Forum [NEAF] Careers group. MCAN aims to support careers advisers who work with medical students and postgraduate doctors, and provides, once a year, a networking day to enable members to share best practice in the provision of career support. NEAF Careers comprises, in the main, staff from Deaneries who have a particular focus on career support. KSS contributes to the work of both MCAN and NEAF Careers, and also benefits from it, particularly from the exchange of ideas for workshops and from the opportunity to share information and resources with other members. This has been helpful in supporting changes to recruitment into Foundation, CST and HST.

# Working with Individual Doctors

Members of the careers team are also available to meet with postgraduate doctors on a referral basis. LEPs can refer a postgraduate doctor if they think they would benefit from further career support. A member of the team is then allocated to the doctor. These meetings are confidential unless the careers adviser has concerns either about the individual's safety or about patient safety, in which case ethical concerns take precedence. A wide range of issues is brought to these discussions – postgraduate doctors may be considering leaving medicine, having difficulty making a career choice, or may wish to request specific help with application forms, CVs, and interviews. From time to time there is also a mentoring aspect to the work, for example, helping individuals to develop the specific skills needed to make particular choices and decisions.

When the adviser first meets someone who has been referred for career support, they will usually spend some time finding out what help that individual needs, and will then design a programme of activities and meetings to meet those needs. Initially, the doctor is usually offered between one and three sessions, although this can be changed as the work continues. There is also flexibility in the system, so that the programme can be amended as required to suit individuals' specific needs. The careers advisers have access to a wide range of exercises, tools, and resources to support this work.

## Working One-to-One: My Own Approach

My work with individuals is underpinned by a number of frameworks. During each session I follow the Ali and Graham model (Ali and Graham 1996; see Figure 4), making sure I start by clarifying my client's goals for the session. We then explore how these goals might be achieved, evaluating ideas and options which have been identified. Finally, the client is asked to devise an action plan. During a session we might move between stages and go back and recontract what needs to be covered. Every session is different and coaching skills are an important contributor to the interaction with the client.

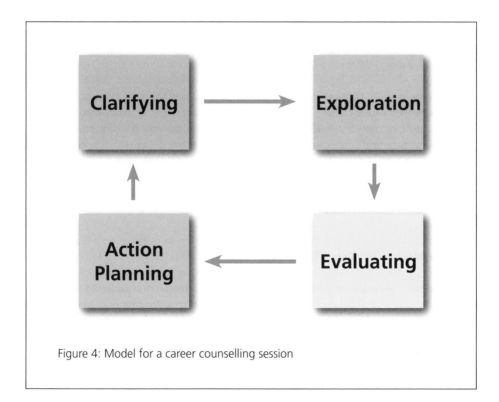

Figure 4: Model for a career counselling session

I trained as a coach in 2000 and became particularly interested in helping people with career choices and decisions. The approach I take with postgraduate doctors uses my skills, knowledge and abilities in coaching, mentoring and career decision making. For me, coaching is 'a human development process which involves structured, focused interaction and use of appropriate strategies, tools and techniques to promote desirable and sustainable change for the benefit of the coachee and potentially for other stakeholders' (Cox et al 2010, 1).

The Cedefop Report referred to above discusses the issue of career skills and career education, and introduces the concept of 'career coaching'. The work I do at KSS falls into this category. The team as a whole aims to develop individuals' career management skills and also to provide LEPs with the information, resources, and education they need to offer career support locally.

My own interest in coaching and mentoring has continued to develop while I have been working at KSS. The usefulness of providing mentoring for doctors after they have made their choices for CST and HST, to aid with their continuing career choices, has been highlighted by a number of writers, including Tooke (2007) and BMA cohort studies. Mentoring to support newly appointed consultants, career-grade doctors, and some specialties, such as General Practice, has also been advocated within the UK. Bristol GP Solutions (in conjunction with the Severn Deanery) runs a successful mentoring scheme for GPs (http://www.bristolgpsolutions. org.uk/) and KSS runs both a co-mentoring scheme for new consultants and a mentoring scheme for GPs. A DH report *Mentoring for Doctors* (2004) positively recommends both mentoring and co-mentoring. It questions the wisdom of offering mentoring only to new consultants: its preference is to look at mentoring as part of continuing career development. More recently French (2007) has written about the mentoring scheme introduced in the East Midlands Healthcare Workforce Deanery.

In KSS, there is an encouraging interest in the use of mentoring to assist postgraduate doctors with their career choices and progression. Agomo (2006) describes how mentoring from a consultant provided much-needed help and support with her career progression, and in the same article proposes that everyone needs a mentor. Certainly all postgraduate doctors would benefit from the opportunity to discuss their career progression issues with someone trained to provide such support.

## Responding to Local Needs

KSS considered a range of theoretical approaches and research in order to develop its system and processes for careers support. Recent research by Bimrose and Barnes (2007) tracked individuals who received guidance interviews and identified a number of career competencies: researching employment and / or course requirements; seeking employment; education and / or training opportunities; understanding labour-market conditions; writing CV and / or job applications; interviewing skills; reflecting with others on options and decisions; demonstrating confidence in career decisions; and good networking and communication skills. These skills are similar in many ways to those we sought to develop through the writing of ROADS (Elton and Reid 2010). Bimrose and Barnes (2007) also reported that guidance was seen to be useful when it challenged ideas and understanding, inspired self-confidence, and increased self-awareness. Access to relevant information and structured opportunities to talk to a professional were also identified as important. It was found that as a result of the guidance they had received, those taking part in the study acquired career resilience and the ability to take charge of their own careers and to manage challenging and difficult circumstances. The changes to medical career pathways have meant that postgraduate doctors require encouragement to gain confidence in understanding and managing their career pathways.

The careers team provides regular drop-in sessions in LEPs where a careers adviser will typically see between five and six doctors for half an hour each. The majority of the doctors who come to these sessions are in Foundation and the issues discussed range from specialty choices to practical help with application forms and interviews. Follow-up sessions are occasionally arranged to handle more in-depth issues. Typically, at any one time, each member of the careers team will be working with two to four clients who have been referred for more in-depth support. The support they require may range from identifying an appropriate career path to considering changing specialty and may include leaving medicine and seeking an alternative career.

In summary, career support in KSS is strongly informed by our recognition that career and learning are linked inextricably, as Cedefop indicates (2008, 13). Because postgraduate doctors are in both employment and education, we have sought to provide a flexible range of approaches through which their career paths and choices can be discussed, including individual and group career conversations, printed resources, and electronic resources. We believe that the location of the careers team within the KSS Education Department provides us with the most advantageous position for supporting postgraduate doctors as they make well-informed and appropriate career choices linked to their PGME.

# References

Agomo, A. 2006. *Mentors – who needs them anyway?* http://careers.bmj.com/careers/advice/view-article.html?id=2001 (accessed January 18, 2011).

Ali, L., and B. Graham. 1996. *The Counselling Approach to Careers Guidance*. London: Routledge.

Arnold, J. 1997. *Managing Careers into the 21st Century*. London: Chapman.

Bimrose, J., and S-A. Barnes. 2007. *Navigating the Labour Market: career decision making and the role of guidance*. University of Warwick: Warwick Institute for Employment Research and Department for Education and Skills.

Borges, N. J., and M. L. Savickas. 2002. Personality and medical specialty choice: a literature review and integration. *Journal of Career Assessment* 3: 362-80.

British Medical Association. 2003. *Signposting medical careers for doctors*. http://www.bma.org.uk//ap.nsf/Content/signposting (accessed January 18, 2011).

British Medical Association. *Cohort Studies*. http://www.bma.org.uk//healthcare_policy/cohort_studies/index.jsp (accessed January 18, 2011).

Cedefop 2008. *Career Development at Work: a review of career guidance to support people in employment*. http://www.cedefop.europa.eu/EN/Files/5183_en.pdf (accessed January 18, 2011).

Cox, E., T. Bachkirova, and D. Clutterbuck. 2010. *The Complete Handbook of Coaching*. London: Sage.

Darzi, A. 2008. *High Quality Care for All: NHS Next Stage Review final report*. Command 7432. London: Department of Health.

*DENI 2009. Preparing for Success: careers education, information, advice and guidance*. www.deni.gov.uk/ceiag_pfs-2.pdf (accessed January 18, 2011).

Department of Health 2004. *Mentoring for Doctors: Signposts to current practice for career grade doctors – guidance from the Doctors' Forum*. http://www.dh.gov.uk/en/Publicationsandstatistics/Publications/PublicationsPolicyAndGuidance/DH_4089395 (accessed January 18, 2011).

Department of Health 2003. *Modernising medical careers: The response of the four UK Health Ministers to the consultation on "Unfinished Business: Proposals for reform of the senior house officer grade"*. http://www.dh.gov.uk/en/Publicationsandstatistics/Publications/PublicationsPolicyAndGuidance/DH_4010460 (accessed January 18, 2011).

Elton, C. 2006. *Helping Foundation Trainees with Their Career Planning: outlining a structured delivery model for The South Thames Foundation Schools*. London KSS Deanery.

Elton, C., and J. Reid. 2010. *ROADS to Success*. 3rd ed. London: KSS Deanery.

French, G. 2007. Mentoring for self development. *National Association of Clinical Tutors UK Bulletin* 44: 2225-2228.

Hall, D. T. 1976. *Careers in Organisations*. Santa Monica: Goodyear.

Hirsh, W., C. Jackson, and J. M. Kidd. 2001. *Straight Talking: effective career discussions at work*. Cambridge: National Institute for Careers Education and Counselling (NICEC).

Jackson, C., J. E. Ball, W. Hirsh, and J. M. Kidd. 2003. *Informing Choices: the need for career advice in medical training*. Cambridge: National Institute for Careers Education and Counselling (NICEC).

Krieshok, T.S., M. D. Black, and R. A. McKay. 2009. Career Decision Making: The limits of rationality and the abundance of non-conscious processes. *Journal of Vocational Behavior* 75: 275-290.

Moss, P.J., T. W. Lambert, M. J. Goldacre, and P. Lee. 2004. Reasons for considering leaving UK medicine: questionnaire study of junior doctors' comments. http://www.bmj.com/content/329/7477/1263.full (accessed January 18, 2011).

Offer, M., and J. P. Sampson Jr. 1999. Quality in the content and use of information and communications technology in guidance. *British Journal of Guidance and Counselling* 27 (4): 501-516.

Oliver, L. W., and S. C. Whiston. 2000. Internet career assessment for the new millennium. *Journal of Career Assessment* 8 (4): 361-369.

Patel, S. G., R. Ahmed, B. P. Rosenbaum, and S. M. Rodgers. 2008. Career guidance and the web: bridging the gap between the AAMC careers in medicine website and local career guidance programs. Teaching and Learning in Medicine 20 (3): 230-234.

Taylor, K., T. Lambert, and M. Goldacre. 2008. Future career plans of a cohort of senior doctors working in the National Health Service. *Journal Royal Society of Medicine* 101: 182-190.

Tooke, J. 2007. *Aspiring to Excellence: final report of the independent inquiry into Modernising Medical Careers*. London: MMC Inquiry.

Turner, G., M. J. Goldacre, T. Lambert, T. and J. W. Sear. 2005. Career choices for anaesthesia: national survey of graduates of 1974-2002 from UK medical schools. *British Journal of Anaesthesia* 95 (3): 332-338.

Watts, A. G. 1999. Reshaping career development for the 21st century. http://www.derby.ac.uk/files/icegs_reshaping_career_development1999a.pdf (accessed January 18, 2011).

# Professionalism, Medical Humanities and the Art of Medicine

Medicine is both an art and a science, the axiom says, locating it firmly in both the humanist and the empirical traditions (Herman 2001). However, the most immediately familiar identity of medical education in the Western intellectual tradition (Tarnas 1991) is as a means of teaching a science, drawing on a technical-rational idea of 'facts' – items of knowledge that are universal, observable, repeatable and, above all, amenable to the 'scientific method' of quantification and verification.

What, then, is the art of medicine? The answer that science lies in the theory of medicine, and that art, therefore, lies in the practice of medicine, is an attractive one, conjuring up an image of gentle scientists using their hard-won, specialist, empirical knowledge to alleviate the suffering of unfortunate humanity, whatever people's rank or creed. This answer should not be neglected, since it points both to the emancipatory purpose of education, and to a role in social justice that lies at the heart of medicine, combining both qualities in the idea of medical education. However, attractive though this idea may be, it should not be taken as an adequate answer. It is problematic to formulate 'medical' as meaning science, theory, and quantity, and to formulate 'education' as meaning art, practice, and quality. First, such a formulation sets up a binary between the two sets of terms, positioning each as exclusive. Second, it suggests that the practice of medicine is secondary to its theory, rather than that both inform each other, as happens in the real-life clinical encounter. Third, it suggests that medicine focuses on only one kind of knowledge – theory, 'knowing that' – a view that does not reflect the actual progress of learners from undergraduate to postgraduate medical education [PGME]. As Chapter 2 discusses, more than one kind of knowledge is needed to learn the practice of medicine, since 'knowing that' must be accompanied by 'knowing how'. Finally, that formulation, and the image of the doctor relieving the pain of the patient, expresses a clear relationship of power, benign power it is true, but still suggestive of the patient as the passive object of the doctor's work. This provides a quite different feeling from the idea that the clinical encounter should be a meeting of doctor and patient for a shared discussion, to a common purpose, as required by two key tenets of the General

Medical Council's [GMC] *Good Medical Practice*: 'Treat patients as individuals and respect their dignity'; and 'Work in partnership with patients' (GMC 2009, frontispiece).

# A Sufficient Curriculum

At the time of writing, understanding the right relationship between the art and science of medicine is more important than ever, since all of the National Curriculum Frameworks [NCFs] for PGME are being rewritten for implementation in Local Education Providers [LEPs] across the whole of the UK. As indicated in Chapter 1, *The Gold Guide* requires that every NCF must contain 'Professionalism', and that every postgraduate doctor must learn and demonstrate 'psychosocial and humanistic qualities such as caring, empathy, humility and compassion, social responsibility and sensitivity to people's culture and beliefs' (MMC 2010, 110). The requirement for professionalism is absolute as far as the GMC is concerned, since the standards set out in *Good Medical Practice* must be adhered to by all doctors, 'whether or not you hold a licence to practise and whether or not you routinely see patients' (GMC 2009, 5). GMC uses the term 'must' in a very particular way, saying '"must" is used for an overriding duty or principle' (GMC 2009, 5) and so the requirements of *Good Medical Practice* have the ethical force of Kant's Categorical Imperative discussed in Chapter 2. This means that curriculum development for medical education is a morally charged activity.

In Kent, Surrey and Sussex Postgraduate Medical Deanery [KSS], we use Stenhouse's (1975, 5) definition of a curriculum:

> The means by which the experience of attempting to put an educational proposal into practice is made publicly available. It involves both content and method, and in its widest application takes account of the problem of implementation.

Stenhouse's requirement is for an explicit curriculum, one that can be made 'publicly available', so that the qualities that comprise 'professionalism' can be understood, discussed, explored, and accounted for. Further, this definition foregrounds the idea of a curriculum arising out of practice, which, as well as being explicit about principles, purposes, content, experiences, outcomes, and processes, also requires explicitness about its ethics, since ethics form a fundamental part of a curriculum statement for clinical practice.

A sufficient curriculum for PGME, therefore, must provide an expression of its whole theory and practice: the art of medicine, as well as its science; professionalism as 'knowing how', as well as 'knowing that'. The KSS approach to developing professionalism, therefore, is to explore what the art of medicine comprises, what tacit understandings about the 'psychosocial and humanistic qualities' of medical practice might be made explicit, and how professionalism might be taught and learned. We believe that these explorations will broaden and deepen practitioners' understandings of their practice, extend important interdisciplinary aspects of the real-life clinical workplace, and provide a means of developing that most elusive of all clinical qualities, 'insight'. Ultimately, of course, professionalism has an immediate and direct patient-safety agenda, and it is with this purpose in mind that KSS and Birkbeck College teach a part-time MA degree in Medical Humanities, to seek new ways of improving patient care, for the new National Health Service [NHS].

Like all other aspects of our work described in this book, the subject of Medical Humanities in KSS begins with the real-life, messy, problematic world of everyday clinical practice, and focuses on improving patient care. It is concerned with local complexity, creativity, and diversity, and thus recognises the interdependency of theory and practice, of art and science, and of humanistic and technical principles, as they arise in usual patient care. It allows the particular person to be understood in the light of universal values, and vice versa since it promotes questions about individual needs, experiences, and understandings, and how they might change in different contexts and circumstances. From this standpoint, patients cease to be objectified as raw material, as passive bodies to be acted on by active scientists. Their intersubjectivity is recognised, that is, they are seen as people, with agency and autonomy, as owners of their bodies and lives, and as having a voice and a choice. Such views intertwine humanism with technology, so that they overlap, illuminate each other, and create a 'third space', an interstitial area, or contact zone, where real-life learning and practice co-construct each other. In curriculum terms, this is the Curriculum in Practice [CiP], that is, the curriculum as it is experienced and created by patients, learners, and teachers, in their processes of creating explicit, mutually agreed roles, responsibilities, boundaries, and expectations.

These ideas, principles, and values have always been held implicitly by Western medicine, communicated in powerful ethical statements such as the Hippocratic Oath, the Oath of Maimonedes, and the Physician's Oath of the World Medical Association. Enmeshed in the inspiring, poetic language of these Oaths are ideas about knowledge, history, intuition, and the imagination – that is, the humanities – and their relationship to patients, doctors, and scientific medicine. Exploring these ideas, and making them available for discussion, is the remit of Medical Humanities.

## Two Kinds of Knowledge

The implication of my opening idea, that the science of medicine lies in the theory, and its art lies in its practice, is that each clinical encounter is a synthesis of theory and practice. In Chapter 2, I describe this as the relationship between part and whole, the logical relationship between the 'necessary' and the 'sufficient', in which the part is contained within the whole, a smaller term contained by a larger term, as a yolk is part of a whole egg. So, the part is necessary, but not sufficient, to describe the whole. These are logical relationships, expressed in Chapter 2 as 'fried egg' diagrams, but shown more formally in logic as a set of analogies. So, the relationship between part and whole is analogous to the relationship between the necessary and the sufficient, usually written as:

**part: whole ↔ necessary: sufficient**

Such a logical relationship is a basic building block of Western philosophy, operating throughout our daily lives, as, for example, the relationship between the particular and the universal, between time and eternity, or between *bios* and *zoe*:

**particular: universal ↔ time: eternity ↔ *bios: zoe***

In terms of different kinds of knowledge – different epistemologies – a similar logical relationship exists between *episteme* and *gnosis*. By *episteme* is meant knowledge of fixed systems, things that stand in a specific, unalterable relationship to each other – mathematics, anatomy, or the laws of the physical universe, for example. *Gnosis* is a different kind of knowledge: it is knowledge arising from relationship, created by different people and things operating together to form a whole, which can be fluid, provisional, changing, and developing. The knowledge arising from relationship includes the knowledge of fixed systems, and so *episteme* as the smaller term is contained by *gnosis* as the larger term, although, of course, *episteme* can never contain *gnosis*. *Episteme* is vitally necessary to medical practice but only *gnosis* is sufficient to describe professionalism's requirement for caring, empathy, humility, compassion, social responsibility, and sensitivity to people's culture and beliefs.

Part of medicine, then – the science, the facts – is *episteme*, but it is held within, and given meaning by, *gnosis* – the understanding of how the science interacts between the patient and doctor, their contexts, the setting, the other people involved, everyone's needs, abilities, and achievements. *Episteme* describes the particular place, time, and sequence of events, but their meaning is created and contained by *gnosis*, the web of relationships, through which the events are understood as having quality and feeling. *Episteme* is created by these factors being brought into context with each other. *Gnosis* supplies the art of medicine, as *episteme* supplies its science: science and technology are necessary to medicine, but not sufficient to describe its whole practice. Expressed logically:

**part: whole ↔ necessary: sufficient ↔ *episteme: gnosis* ↔ science: art**

# Two Kinds of History

In the Western mind's collective narrative of events, *episteme* appears as history, in the form of a detailing of recorded, verifiable facts, gathered and interpreted by careful historians. These are used to make increasingly complete accounts, from a range of perspectives, working in the tradition of *episteme* to provide a detailed, balanced, complex narrative of the past. However, such historical accounts are always partial, both in the sense of being a record of only a part of what happened, and in the sense of providing a particular viewpoint, since proverbially, history is written by the victors. Furthermore, because this task of *episteme* is an important and engaging one, it is dominant in our understanding of the term 'history', and thus it can be easy to overlook history as *gnosis*. *Gnosis* is history as a set of strong, recurrent relationships, not just between people and other people, but between people and the whole world they occupy. It supplies a sacred history – 'sacred' means literally, 'making whole' – the literature, arts, music, landscapes, buildings, and artefacts that express a culture's mythology, the *zoe* of the individual *bios*: life out of time, rather than life-in-time, the meaning of life as an absolute value.

This is important to medicine, where reverberant symbols of a staff with two snakes and a staff with one snake, speak to its sacred ancestry. The staff with one snake is an attribute of Asklepios, teacher of Hippocrates, himself taught by the centaur Chiron, who received the sacred knowledge from Apollo. It indicates medicine's life-in-time, its *bios*, a genealogical inscription, traced through a line of inheritance, as a traditionally historic, sequential account. For medicine's *zoe*, the eternal, categorical valuing of human life, that is fundamental to clinical ethics and practice, it is necessary to go to the caduceus, the staff with two snakes, which is an attribute of Hermes, and which indicates the liminal positioning of doctors, literally at the borderline between life and death. Of all the Olympic pantheon, only Hermes can travel between Hades, the dark realm of death, and the everyday world of light and life. Mythologically, then, both Apollo and Hermes are needed to represent the whole of medicine's work and realm, both the single and the double snakes, the *bios* and the *zoe*. Indeed, as the Homeric *Hymn to Hermes* makes clear, the two gods are brothers (Cashford 2003, 55-84).

Unsurprisingly, then, 'health' also means 'whole', from the Anglo-Saxon 'hale', and in order to 'make whole', the first hospitals were places that evoked eternal values – temples to Asklepios, since 'temple' arises from the root 'tempus', meaning 'time', so that 'temple' is literally 'out of time', in eternity, where *bios* returns to *zoe*, to be restored to wholeness. The literal meaning of these words has been lost, or has declined to denote some kind of superstition, but their resonances are still present. Today, too, as for thousands of years in Western Europe, to enter a hospital is to seek to be made whole, in a place that is outside the usual constraints of daily time, surrendering to life and death possibilities, asking for help from people whose exceptional practice positions them every day on that chthonic borderline – doctors, the priests of Asklepios – and hoping for health, for wholeness, for the literal sacredness of their life to be restored.

History as *gnosis*, then, expresses and arises out of a view of the world as entire and whole – it is a 'sufficient' view. It reflects what the poet W. B. Yeats called the 'Spiritus Mundi' (1950, 211), the life of the world, which his contemporary, psychologist Carl Jung referred to as 'the collective unconscious'. As the literary critic Northrop Frye puts it (1982, xviii):

> Man lives, not directly or nakedly in nature like the animals, but within a mythological universe, a body of assumptions and beliefs developed from his existential concerns. Most of this is held unconsciously, which means that our imaginations may recognize elements of it when presented in art or literature, without consciously understanding what it is that we recognize.

Frye thus distinguishes between 'Weltgeschichte', or history of the material world, and 'Heilgeschichte', the sacred history, which enables us to locate our felt experiences within the larger 'mythological universe'. Similarly, the religious historian Mircea Eliade describes both 'knowledge in the modern sense of the term, objective and compartmentalized information, subject to indefinite correction and addition', and '"sacred history" – mythology [which] is exemplary, paradigmatic: not only does it relate how things came to be; it also lays the foundation for all human behaviour and all social and cultural institutions' (1958, x-xi). These distinctions parallel Jung's 'two kinds of thinking': 'directed thinking', which he sees as exemplified by science and technology, and 'subjective thinking', 'actuated by inner motives . . . based on instinct', through which directed thinking 'is brought into contact with the oldest layers of the human mind, long buried beneath the threshold of consciousness' (Jung 1967, 7-33). In a similar formulation, feminist historian Diane Purkiss (1996) discusses *herstory*, history as affinity, which foregrounds the personal and emotional, in order to interpret and understand the felt, imaginative significance of recorded 'fact'. This distinction is crucially necessary to human consciousness since, as Cashford (2003, 11), succinctly points out, 'the world is not given us as fact but inhabited through interpretation'. Thus, as Martin Buber suggests, experience must be understood both as 'the events themselves', and 'the manner in which the participating people experienced those events' (1946, 16). Cashford quotes Einstein's sombre warning, made in 1964, of the penalties of not reaching for these new understandings: 'The unleashing of the power of the atom bomb has changed everything except our mode of thinking, and thus we head towards unparalleled catastrophes' (2003, 11).

It is crucially important to professionalism, therefore, to recognise that every patient has two histories, one contained in the other, as the part is contained in the whole, and as *episteme* is contained by *gnosis*. The patient's first, immediate history is their *bios*, absolutely necessary for treatment, a partial account of their life-in-time: age, sex, clinical history, injury, condition. This technical view of the patient, caught in a particular moment in time, focuses them as science, and identifies them by injury, so they become 'a fracture', 'an MI', or 'an overdose'. This is the *episteme* of the matter, but it is not the *gnosis* of the person, or of any of the people present, whether labelled as patient, doctor, nurse, patient's family, specialist registrar, ward clerk, or any other technical identity. The *gnosis*, the wholeness of each person, lies in their story, or mythology, in their personal experience of the universal, the affinities that have opened to them in their whole, 'sacred' history: the beliefs, views, feelings, perceptions, and ideas through which they inhabit the world. Succinctly, strong *episteme* is necessary, but only *gnosis* is sufficient for 'a whole team' to treat 'the whole patient' as part of an organisational 'whole systems' approach. The art of medicine lies in developing that *gnosis*, at every level of patient care.

## Intuition, Imagination and Science

Science, of course, has always been aware of this 'other world' of artistic, imaginative truth. Even as Newton formulated his magisterially universal laws of gravity and thermodynamics, and ushered in the scientific revolution, he was working also as a noted alchemist, concerned with the alchemical quest for the philosopher's stone, spiritual perfection, expressed as the ability to turn base metal into gold. As Harpur (2002, 163-4) points out, in their search for 'the union of the four elements, Mercurius quadruplex', alchemists referred to their work variously as 'our art, our science, and our philosophy', so that it is unsurprising to find Newton, at the end of his life, couching the relationship between his scientific and his metaphysical searches in terms of part and whole, reportedly saying (Brewster 1855, 407):

> I do not know what I may appear to the world, but to myself I seem to have been only like a boy playing on the sea-shore, and diverting myself in now and then finding a smoother pebble or a prettier shell than ordinary, whilst the great ocean of truth lay all undiscovered before me.

Newton's contemporary, the visionary poet and painter William Blake, sought actively to reconcile *episteme* and *gnosis* through his art, pointing to the need for 'a double vision' (*CW* 816-8), and commenting:

> Every body does not see alike. . . The tree which moves some to tears of joy is in the Eyes of others only a Green thing that stands in the way. Some See Nature all Ridicule & Deformity . . . & Some Scarce see Nature at all. But to the Eyes of the Man of Imagination, Nature is Imagination itself. As a man is, So he Sees. As the Eye is formed, such are its Powers (*CW* 793).

In their different ways, both Newton the physicist and Hermetic alchemist, and Blake the poet and painter, were working within the same enduring philosophy, Neo-Platonism, which Raine (1979, 2-3) says:

> may be compared to an underground river that flows through European history, sending up, from time to time, springs and fountains; and wherever its fertilizing stream emerges, there imaginative thought revives, and we have a period of great art and poetry. The works that taught Blake and the other English Romantic poets are the same that inspired the Florentine School of Athens, the American Transcendentalists, and in our own time laid the foundations of the Irish renaissance; many of the works Blake studied are on the shelves of William Butler Yeats's library, in Dublin, to this day.

In scientific practice, intuition and imagination act as a single, concurrent movement. Intuition, the knowing that comes before knowledge, prompts the scientist to notice a particular item at a particular time: it is, perhaps, the coming together of a lifetime's conscious and unconscious assimilation of knowledge, skills, and experience, to provide an inner prompting, to give particular attention to a particular detail. Concurrently, imagination paints a picture – an *imago*, or image – of what that intuitively perceived detail might, or could, represent or lead to. Suddenly, the whole of the person's power of inquiry is engaged in new discovery. These discoveries are inspired, we say, meaning, literally, that the *inspiro*, the 'breath of the god', has entered and moved the individual: a well-spring of previously unknown ideas has been tapped. It is in this way that Alexander Fleming intuitively noticed and imaginatively visualised the possibilities for penicillin, that Wilhelm Röntgen was inspired to discover x-rays, and that James Watson accounted for the breakthrough that led him to understand the structure of DNA. Similarly, in a contemporary scientific account (Association of Medical Humanities 2010, 12):

> In 2005, Francis Wells, a consultant heart surgeon at Papworth Hospital, Cambridge pioneered repair to damaged hearts from viewing Leonardo's medical drawing derived from dissections. Francis used the drawings to work out how to restore normal opening and closing function of the mitral valve, so that instead of repairing a floppy valve by narrowing its diameter - thereby restricting blood flow under exertion - he underwent 'a complete rethink of the way we do the mitral valve operation' . . . Francis Wells has completed over 2,000 mitral valve repairs, achieving a near 100% rate for fixing leaking mitral valves.

It is significant, perhaps, that Wells's guide, Leonardo, was a member of the Neo-Platonic Florentine Academy, established by Lorenzo de' Medici, poet and statesman, and led by Marsilio Ficino, a doctor's son like Aristotle, the first translator of Plato's works into Latin, in touch with all the great European minds of science, art and philosophy, and a leading humanist of his day.

## Arts and Sciences Resolved

Newtonian science, and even Einstein's physics, have long since given way to quantum physics, in which light is both a wave and a particle, observation of any phenomenon alters it, and the number of dimensions has expanded to ten, or some say eleven, depending on the mathematical theory in play. The multiple vision that Blake found in the natural world has been rediscovered in the laboratory, as Thomas Kuhn, writing about the structure of scientific revolutions in 1968, said it would be reworked and re-envisioned. Kuhn coined the term 'a paradigm shift' to describe the tiny changes in perception, that mean that a whole scientific vision changes utterly, so that the Sun no longer orbits the Earth, atoms become divisible, and the Earth a self-organising entity. At the same time, the post-modern turn, and complexity theory, have elaborated Blake's axiom that 'as a man is, so he sees', through its recognition that complex systems are essentially intersubjective networks of relationships – Newton's 'great ocean of truth' or *gnosis*. Indeed, Lovelock's Gaia Theory (1979), coupled with real and present political concerns about global warming, suggests that working within that complex web of relationships – participating in *gnosis* – may be a matter of personal and species survival.

It is a loss of innocence that every responsible science, perhaps, has to undergo. Nevertheless, recognising the limitations of a purely technical-rational approach also offers an opportunity for science to re-acquaint itself with the larger world of which it is part, to learn to work within the ambiguities, uncertainties and possibilities that characterise the Humanities, which science is rediscovering in itself. In practice, this means learning to work with what Keats called 'Negative Capability'. In a letter to his brothers on 21 December 1817 he said:

> Browne & Dilke walked with me & back from the Christmas pantomime. I had not a dispute but a disquisition with Dilke, on various subjects; several things dovetailed in my mind, & at once it struck me, what quality went to form a Man of Achievement especially in Literature & which Shakespeare possessed so enormously - I mean Negative Capability, that is when a man is capable of being in uncertainties, Mysteries, doubts, without any irritable reaching after fact & reason (Rollins 1958, 193).

The occasion is not a formal discussion or lecture, but an informal, opportunistic conversation – a 'professional conversation', as we call it in KSS. In PGME, this is the process and point of transformation, the moment when the learner suddenly 'gets it', when the words and notes are heard together as a song – it is 'anagogy' as the Renaissance mind termed it, the education of the learner by sudden insight. Every experienced clinician is familiar with this experience: the case in which all the objective data, the *episteme*, clearly point in one direction, but about which a nagging uncertainty enters the mind, unwilled. These doubts and uncertainties have no rational basis – their genesis is instinctive – but if they are followed appropriately, then they lead to knowledge that can throw a new and different light on the case, to the benefit of patient and doctor. Where 'pedagogy' means teacher-led learning, and 'andragogy' means self-directed learning, 'anagogy' means 'led from above', that is, led onto an unexpected path, by a visible fact that reveals an invisible truth. Anagogy and negative capability are part of the formation and practice of doctors, as greatly powerful as they are generally unacknowledged.

It is crucial to note, however, that negative capability requires one to sit within the mysteries, doubts and uncertainties, without an irritable search for an answer. Real-life clinical practice does not operate to a technical-rational model, in which the answer arrives after a pre-ordained period of analysis, any more than the resolution of a patient's condition occurs at a specific point in time, still less a predictable one. Rather, both are a longer-term, gradual shifting of understandings, as every Intensivist knows. In Intensive Treatment Units, patients progress from being monitored minute by minute, to being monitored hour by hour, then day by day, at an individual rate, over an unpredictable time period. Ripeness is all. A point arrives when the learner understands, when resolution has been achieved, when the patient is well, but these are not foreknown, and even in retrospect, they may be difficult to describe. As T. S. Eliot puts it in *Four Quartets* (2001,5):

> I can only say, *there* we have been: but I cannot say where.
> And I cannot say, how long, for that is to place it in time.

Above all, the Humanities provide – restore, really – an additional way of *seeing*. Science's love affair with the microscope, telescope, and every other kind of scope, produced astonishing, breathtaking benefits to humanity, but it also moved medicine's gaze from the personal standpoints and lived experience of individual people. In medicine, the scientific gaze became a Foucauldian 'regarde', penetrating beneath the skin, into humanity as biology and biochemistry, not into people as whole, contextualised individuals. For medicine, therefore, the present shift in science's claims for objectivity is not so much a loss, as a restoration of a newly understood subjectivity: intersubjectivity, the co-construction of a shared narrative about an individual's condition, treatment, and outcome. Such a narrative engages all stakeholders – doctor, patient, team, and organisation: social sciences and management sciences join biomedical sciences to become part of an essentially humanistic project, requiring humanistic insights.

These humanistic insights, and a restored way of seeing, may be learned from the complex accounts of human emotions, actions, and relationships that comprise literature; from the intensely personal possibilities, choices, and consequences depicted by drama; from the nuanced aesthetics involved in art and music's depictions of people, places, and worlds; and from the complex intertwining of mythologies, artefacts, values, and rituals, through which cultures articulate themselves. Experiencing them is to experience, *par excellence*, the 'uncertainties, Mysteries, doubts' of negative capability, and their appreciation requires patience, a slow unfolding, without 'irritable reaching after fact & reason'. It is the same discipline that is required from our Intensivist, or from any clinician faced with a complex and critical case, since the art of medicine is an entry into the world of artistry, where keen observation, alertness to possibilities, provisional judgement, a readiness to notice new information or ideas, receptiveness to ambiguity, and a deep pleasure in weaving these elements together to form many-layered interpretations, and to derive a whole understanding, is required.

## Back to the Future

To return to Raphael's image of Plato and Aristotle, invoked in Chapter 2, what is required is a marriage of art and science, an overlapping, as Plato's and Aristotle's figures overlap, to produce a 'third space', a new location, where apparent contraries are reconciled. It is not a matter of 'either-or', but of 'both'.

Raphael has made this clear in his painting, with a little in-joke, painting Plato's mobile figure as barefoot, a direct reference to the *Symposium*, in which five people, including a doctor, debate the nature of the highest good, the greatest love, and the finest knowledge. In that dialogue, Socrates recounts what he was taught by his own teacher, 'Diotima of Mantinea, a woman wise in this and in many other kinds of knowledge'. Diotima teaches Socrates that in all things that appear antithetical, there is always 'a mean between the two', a third space (*Symposium* § 201-2). Raphael's visual allusion is to Diotima's personification of the lover of wisdom, who, occupying this third space, 'is always poor . . . and has no shoes, nor a house to dwell in; on the bare earth exposed he lies under the open heaven', and yet is also 'bold, enterprising, strong, a mighty hunter . . . keen in the pursuit of wisdom, fertile in resources, a philosopher at all times' (§ 203). This third space is fluid, like the painting's mobile harmonisation of movement, direction, and epistemology, which Raphael suggests by overlapping Plato's and Aristotle's figures. Diotima says, 'that which is always flowing in is always flowing out', so that the third space occupies a kind of homeostasis, since it 'is never in want and never in wealth'. Furthermore, its understandings are always provisional, since it 'is a mean between ignorance and knowledge' (§ 203-4).

As the contemporary French philosopher, Luce Irigaray, points out, Diotima's teaching provides a particular kind of dialectic, since 'it doesn't use opposition to make the first term pass into the second in order to achieve a synthesis of the two . . . she presents, uncovers, unveils the insistence of a third term that is already there and that permits progression: from poverty to wealth, from ignorance to wisdom' (Irigaray 1993, 20). There is, therefore, no requirement for science to exist at the expense of art, or vice versa, where both are oppositional cultures: they are not a battle between competing interests, as writers such as C. P. Snow (1960) suggest. Rather, they are a conversation informed by two perspectives, which are inextricably intertwined at the level of patient care and practice, and together called professionalism.

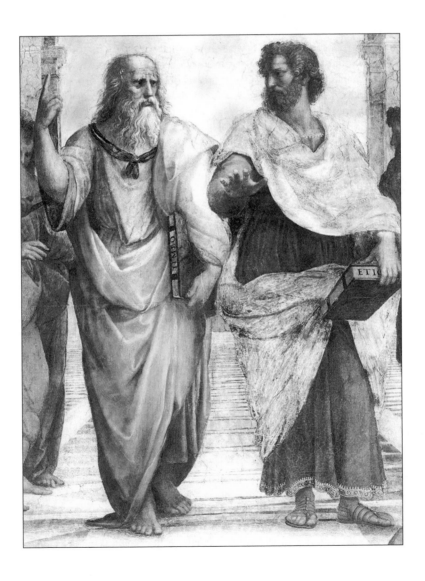

Such a reconciliation of art and science is ever-present but not automatically accessible: it must be sought, as a particular vision. Diotima calls this vision 'daemonic', that is, 'intermediate between the divine and the mortal' (§ 202), since 'daemon' means, literally, 'guardian spirit', which in the context of professionalism we might call 'insight' or 'compassion', or 'conscience', or 'ethical awareness'. Elsewhere, Plato reminds us of the importance to the individual of exercising this 'daemonic' faculty, with a word-play on the Greek for 'happy': 'because he has always looked after the divine element in himself and kept his guardian spirit (*daemon*) in good order he must be happy (*eudaimon*) above all men' (*Timaeus*, 121). For Irigaray (1993, 27), the daemonic is 'a perpetual journey, a perpetual transvaluation, a permanent becoming', that is, it is provisional, highly contextualised, dependent on individual factors, rooted in radical uncertainty, and thus in PGME, co-constructed, patient by patient.

These kinds of epistemologies are being rediscovered by the contemporary Western mind, but for many Indigenous peoples they have never been lost. As Battiste and Henderson (2000, 35) point out, 'most Indigenous scholars choose to view every way of life from two different but complementary perspectives: first as a manifestation of human knowledge, heritage and consciousness, and second as a mode of ecological order'. They enlarge on this to say (2000, 45):

> The traditional ecological knowledge of Indigenous peoples is scientific, in the sense that it is empirical, experimental, and systematic. It differs in two important respects from Western science, however: traditional ecological knowledge is highly localized and it is social. Its focus is the web of relationships between humans, animals, plants, natural forces, spirits, and land forms in a particular locality, as opposed to the discovery of universal "laws." It is the original knowledge of Indigenous peoples. Indigenous peoples have accumulated extraordinarily complex models of species interactions over centuries within very small geographical areas, and they are reluctant to generalize beyond their direct fields of experience. Western scientists, by contrast, concentrate on speculating about and then testing global generalizations, with the result that they know relatively little about the complexities of specific, local ecosystems.

Indigenous knowledge focuses, therefore, on the individual and on the particular, the complex, the uncertain, and the provisional, and on the relationships – we might say, the *gnosis* – that binds these things together, in a particular way, at a particular point in time. Within that 'web of relationships', precision and certainty are generated by empirical observations 'over centuries', but this Indigenous *episteme* is to be understood only within the context of *gnosis*, and not generalised beyond that field of experience. For Battiste and Henderson (2000, 43), Indigenous thought admits 'no separation of science, art, religion, philosophy, or aesthetics'. I suggest that, similarly, recognising the interpenetration of art and science is a precondition to teaching insight and professionalism in PGME.

In real-life practice, each patient arrives with their own story and identity that, as Balint (1957) puts it, they 'offer' to their doctor. To achieve 'sensitivity to people's cultures and beliefs', requires doctor and patient to work from their own personal understanding of the world and to create between them a third space, occupied by *gnosis*, the knowledge formed by relationship. Otherwise, the patient is dehumanised and, instantly, the doctor is deprofessionalised: both become 'cyborgs' (Haraway 1991), both are degraded. The role in social justice, that lies at medicine's heart, is lost: all quality is gone, and doctors are reduced to competent technicians, and patients to raw material, on a production-line NHS. At the level of individual doctor and patient, therefore, good medical practice, and best patient experience, require a humanistic approach.

Further, the Crisp Report on *Global Health Partnerships* (2007) expresses a strong concern that 'Northern' scientific medicine, as it is presently conceived, is not sufficient to create effective partnerships with non-European cultures. This concern is supported by Battiste and Henderson's description of an epistemology that is different from the contemporary 'Eurocentric' approach of biomedicine, providing a different kind of science – more thoughtful, more specific, strongly culturally situated, holistic in the widest sense. At the level of nation, and of the NHS, therefore, there is an increasing discomfort with competing epistemologies.

The purpose of this chapter is to indicate a third space, in which a fuller sense of professionalism may be developed. Deprofessionalisation, degradation, and conflict are not inevitable, neither for individual practitioners and patients, nor for the NHS. Medicine's inheritance is a humanistic tradition, two and a half thousand years old at least, and, although it may have been somewhat overlooked in the remarkable flurry made by science in the two hundred years since Jenner, it is still present. It is a tradition which is still vital and living in Indigenous epistemologies, and its principles are still crucial to defining good medical practice. Called 'professionalism', taught sometimes as 'bedside manner', 'the patient encounter', or 'the consultation', it is what is meant by the 'art of medicine': the disciplines, inquiries and waymarks studied as Medical Humanities. Exploring this re-discovered stream of professional artistry opens up, for the medical profession, wider and deeper understandings of their work, and waymarks a route to creating a more nuanced and richer sense of medical professionalism.

# References

Association of Medical Humanities. 2010. The heart of Leonardo da Vinci decoded: current directions. *Humanities at the Cutting Edge*. Plymouth: Peninsula College of Medicine and Dentistry.

Balint, M. 1957. *The Doctor, His Patient and the Illness*. London: Churchill Livingstone.

Battiste, M. & Henderson, J. Y. 2000. *Protecting Indigenous Knowledge and Heritage*. Saskatoon Saskatchewan, Canada: Punch.

Blake, W. 1972. *Complete Writings*. Ed. Geoffrey Keynes. London: Oxford University Press.

Brewster, D. 1855. *Memoirs of the Life, Writings and Discoveries of Sir Isaac Newton*. Vol. 2. Edinburgh: Thomas Constable & Co.

Buber, M. 1946. *Moses*. Oxford: East and West.

Cashford, J. 2003. *The Homeric Hymns*. London: Penguin.

Crisp, N. 2007. *Global Health Partnerships*. London: COI

Eliade, M. 1958. *Rites and Symbols of Initiation*. New York: Harper.

Eliot, T. S. 2001. (First published 1944). *Four Quartets*. London: Faber and Faber.

Frye, N. 1982. *The Great Code: The Bible and Literature*. London: Routledge & Kegan Paul.

General Medical Council. 2009. *Good Medical Practice*. London: GMC.

Haraway, D. 1991. The Cyborg Manifesto:Science, Technology, and Socialist-Feminism in the Late Twentieth Century. *Simians, Cyborgs and Women: The Prevention of Nature*. New York: Routledge.

Harpur, P. 2002. *The Philosopher's Secret Fire*. London: Penguin.

Herman, J. 2001. Medicine: the science and the art. *Medical Humanities*. 27: 42-46.

Irigaray, L. 1993. *An Ethics of Sexual Difference*. Translated by Carolyn Burke and Gillian C. Gill. London: Athlone.

Plato. 1892. Symposium. *The Dialogues of Plato*. Vol. 1. Translated by B. Jowett. Oxford: Clarendon Press.

Plato. 1971. Timaeus. *Timaeus and Critias*. Translated by Desmond Lee and edited by Betty Radice. London: Penguin.

Jung, C. G. 1967. (First published 1956). *Symbols of Transformation*. New York: Princeton University Press.

Kuhn, T. S. 1968. *The Structure of Scientific Revolutions*. Chicago: University of Chicago Press.

Lovelock, J. 1979. *Gaia*. Oxford: Oxford University Press.

Modernising Medical Careers (MMC). 2010. *A Reference Guide for Postgraduate Specialty Training in the UK: The Gold Guide*. 4th edition. London: NHS.

Purkiss, D. 1996. *The Witch in History*. London: Routledge.

Raine, K. 1979. *Blake and Antiquity*. London: Routledge and Kegan Paul.

Rollins, H. E. 1958. *The Letters of John Keats,1814-1821*. Vol. 1. Cambridge: University Press.

Ryle, G. (1949). *The Concept of Mind*. London, Hutchinson.

Snow, C. P. 1960. *The Two Cultures*. Cambridge: University Press.

Stenhouse, L. 1975. *An Introduction to Curriculum Research and Development*. London: Heinemann Educational.

Tarnas, R. 1991. *The Passion of the Western Mind*. New York: Ballantine Books.

Yeats, W. B. 1950. *Collected Poems*. London: Macmillan.